Speaking Up

....

Understanding Language and Gender

Allyson Jule

MULTILINGUAL MATTERS
Bristol • Blue Ridge Summit

DOI https://doi.org/10.21832/jule9603

Library of Congress Cataloging in Publication Data

A catalog record for this book is available from the Library of Congress.
Names: Jule, Allyson – author.
Title: Speaking Up: Understanding Language and Gender/Allyson Jule.
Description: Bristol; Blue Ridge Summit, PA: Multilingual Matters, 2018. |
Includes bibliographical references and index.
Identifiers: LCCN 2017059873| ISBN 9781783099597 (pbk: alk. paper) |
ISBN 9781783099603 (hbk: alk. paper) | ISBN 9781783099634 (kindle)
Subjects: LCSH: Communication—Sex differences. | Sexism in language.
Classification: LCC P96.S48 J685 2018 | DDC 408.1—dc23 LC record
available at https://lccn.loc.gov/2017059873

British Library Cataloguing in Publication Data

A catalogue entry for this book is available from the British Library.

ISBN-13: 978-1-78309-960-3 (hbk)
ISBN-13: 978-1-78309-959-7 (pbk)

Multilingual Matters

UK: St Nicholas House, 31-34 High Street, Bristol BS1 2AW, UK.
USA: NBN, Blue Ridge Summit, PA, USA.

Website: www.multilingual-matters.com
Twitter: Multi_Ling_Mat
Facebook: https://www.facebook.com/multilingualmatters
Blog: www.channelviewpublications.wordpress.com

The policy of Multilingual Matters/Channel View Publications is to use papers that
are natural, renewable and recyclable products, made from wood grown in
sustainable forests. In the manufacturing process of our books, and to further
support our policy, preference is given to printers that have FSC and PEFC Chain of
Custody certification. The FSC and/or PEFC logos will appear on those books where
full certification has been granted to the printer concerned.

Typeset by Nova Techset Private Limited, Bengaluru and Chennai, India.
Printed and bound in the UK by the CPI Books Group Ltd.

Speaking Up

About the Author

Allyson Jule is an academic specialising in the interaction between language and gender. She is Co-Director of the Gender Studies Institute and Professor of Education at Trinity Western University, Canada. She is also an associate of the University of Oxford's International Gender Studies Centre. She has published widely, and her work has been featured in TIME magazine and The Ladies Home Journal.

Dedicated to all who care about creating a more just world.

'This is not your fault, but it is your problem'.

Alex Bilmes, Editor-in-Chief,
Esquire, March 2016: 126

Contents

. . . .

Prologue

. . . .

The world has changed a great deal over the past few years on a wide range of geopolitical realities as well as on gender issues. For example, less than a decade ago, little attention was paid to transgenderism, but there is now significant discussion on the issue. There have also been an increasing number of conversations in the West concerning diversity, including gender related ones, such as the use of the veil among Muslim communities. How gender is a part of religious communities, including Islamic communities, was not on the radar twenty-years ago. Much more attention is being given to the notion of the continuum of gender identity in various settings, including in schools and as revealed and lived out on social media relations with the steady changes in technology opening up new contexts for gender. There have been various public awareness campaigns like *Ban Bossy, I am a Girl* and Emma Watson's *HeforShe* reveal how public discourse has shifted more towards the connecting of language and gender than ever before. And 2018's #Metoo and #TimesUp movements have altered the way Hollywood recognizes sexual harassment. It seems the world has caught on to the power of language in meaning-making and in framing gender/sexual identities and relationships.

We are so much more aware of gender as a key variable in who and what we are and, specifically the concern here, in how we use language to inhabit our spaces and places. It is now well understood that everyone needs to work together to make the kind of world that is just and sustainable for all of us. Catherine Redfern and Kristin Aune (2013) discuss the developing *new feminism* that is attracting fresh and vibrant young people to the field. British actor Emma Watson is an example of a vibrant and engaged new feminist, and the #Metoo generation has moved feminism along to a new accountability regarding sexism in the workplace. More and more young people are engaging with the field after what has seemed to be a period of apathy that expressed a kind of 'battle fatigue' concerning feminism throughout the 1990s and early 2000s. The stakes seem higher than ever as we face yet more complexity related to how gender issues fit into some of the world's most pressing problems: a major shift in American politics to the right; increase awareness of sexual harassment by (often) men in positions of power; Islamic terrorism and violence; the refugee crisis; gender-based violence on university campuses and in conflict zones; increasing poverty in developing countries; shifts in geo-political alliances; climate change; assaults on Western democracies; and the continued and even greater risk for girls and young women seeking an education in many areas of the world where their participation is limited. It is because of these concerns and the rise of new and compelling feminist concerns that many writers such as Redfern and Aune see a 'new excitement in the feminist movement which seems to be growing exponentially' (2013: x).

This book is designed to be an accessible introduction to academic research in this dynamic field. So much of what we hear from others or read about in magazines or hear about on talk shows is other people's opinions, and other people's opinions do not really reflect current research on a whole assortment of gender and language contexts. Spoken language use and gender as a social variable intersect in the key contexts in which we live our lives, such as in the media, in schools, in the workplace, in religious communities and within family life.

Speaking Up: Understanding Language and Gender is an exploration of the ever-widening research area of gender and language use and the changes in many communities regarding gender equity issues. It is my hope to encourage those with interest in these issues to understand some of the past and current complexities surrounding gender and language and to consider some new directions that are already becoming increasingly clear. In many parts of the world, language remains a key tool of oppression used to ensure that (often powerless) women and sexual minorities do not share power equally with white heterosexual men. I believe that if we can make hidden assumptions about gender and language more explicit, then we can play a part in making this world a better place to live as human beings. Also, such is the pace of change in these areas that this book is a snapshot of current thought. Who would have imagined the reality of a Trump presidency a few years ago? One cannot miss the connection of gender and language watching America under Trump: for example, the way he dismissed his opponent, Hillary Clinton, and other women, mocking a woman's appearance and discarding women's voices entirely. As his presidency goes on, I suspect there will be more examples of how language is used to limit the involvement and contributions of others in positions of power and how gender identity shapes beliefs and attitudes and, language use. In such ways, I see gender, sexuality and language continuing to shift alongside the study of gender, sexuality and language. In my opinion, this study will continue to be one of the most compelling areas of study around the world. I hope you will agree.

Allyson Jule
Vancouver, BC
Canada

I

Understanding Gender and Language Use

. . . .

1

The Basics

. . . .

I don't know why people are so reluctant to say they're feminists.
Could it be any more obvious that we still live in a patriarchal world
when 'feminism' is a bad word?

Ellen Page

Gender roles and behaviors have interested me my whole life. I grew up with an older brother and sister and, like everyone else, my early life experiences were heavily influenced by the sex I was born with. In my cultural context, this meant that I had a pink bedroom and was absolutely delighted to receive Barbie dolls for Christmas. My mother was a nurse, a good cook and an attentive homemaker; my father 'went to work', cut the grass and took care of the car. In short, I grew up with stereotypical gender modeling around me. Until I came to recognize the assumptions embedded within the gender distinctions that these models presented, I saw being a girl as unproblematic. After all, I liked Barbie dolls – as did my sister. We felt no oppression. My life goal to be a language teacher seemed very possible and realistic. Without extraordinary effort, I qualified as a teacher in due course. In many ways I am a 'typical' woman: I am married to a man, I have children, I like to decorate and read, and I have chosen a profession easily open to women: education. Would these realities have been the same had I been born male or not straight? Perhaps. Likely not.

The lived realities of being female, feminine, male or masculine is central here in relation to language use. There are two reasons why I am writing this book on gender and language use. One is that being formed, rehearsed and rewarded by my culture into performances of gender and gendered life choices predicts lives like mine. This universal human reality (that we are deeply connected to our communities through our genderedness) is in and of itself reason enough to consider the complexities and the implications of gender. The second reason is that rehearsals into genderedness are most fascinatingly revealed in language use, language tendencies and language patterns. An interest in the relationship of language use and one's gender emerged from my experiences as a classroom language teacher. I noticed over the years that the boys and girls in my classrooms were having quite distinct experiences and were preparing for different possibilities for future experiences.

One example of gendered tendencies as expressed in language use is the way I have begun to write this book. I have already used a gendered tendency by using personal anecdote. This is the writing 'voice' I am most comfortable using. Why might this be? Apparently, this personal revelation style is something understood by my society as 'feminine' because it is viewed as relatable and accessible. (In 1990, Deborah Tannen identified this as 'relational' talk.) This relational style might serve my purposes here quite well – to draw you in by making you feel a personal connection; or it might limit my authority by undermining the legitimacy of what I might have to say. In other words, this style interacts with each reader in a unique way. But regardless, my performance of gender and its particular recognition by you, the reader, matters a great deal to my message: how we speak reveals our gendered tendencies, and it also continues to perpetuate these tendencies. Your reaction to this style of relational writing tells us something about you, too. You might expect me to write in a certain way because I am an academic. Importantly, these gendered roles have less to do with which sex we were born with and more to do with our surrounding society's values, norms, and expectations of each sex.

In this book, I seek to introduce you to the exciting world of language use (both its powers and its limitations) through and with the lens of gendered expectations. My hope is that this beginner's guide will be accessible as well as engaging for you, and that it will inspire you to continue to explore and reflect on the ways gender identities impact our communication and how our language use impacts our performances of gender. Gender is a major part of who we are and why we behave in certain ways, and so it is worthwhile to consider the many places that gender and language intersect. This first chapter addresses the development of the academic field known as 'Gender, Sexuality and Language'. What follows is a discussion of key concepts and terminology used in the field.

Feminism: A Quick Review

The *Oxford English Dictionary* defines feminism as 'the policy, practice, or advocacy of the political, economic and social equality for women'. This definition is helpful enough but there are strong connotations around the word 'feminism' that a dictionary definition cannot adequately explore. Today's feminism is a diverse phenomenon with a very long history. The current field includes three main camps:

1. *Liberal feminism* which seeks primarily to watch and comment on society's portrayal of women as indicative of society's patriarchal attitudes and values.
2. *Socialist feminism* which sees patriarchy alongside social class issues of dominance and power and in need of challenge.
3. *Radical feminism* which views women as oppressed and seeks to challenge power relations that exist between women and men.

Intersectional feminism is also important to understand because of the various identities we all have, including our gender, sexual identity as well as race, social class, nationality, socio-economic status, etc.

This book comes from a liberal feminist position because its main aim is to comment on society's portrayal of gender. Other variations include, among many others, psychoanalytic feminism, queer feminism, postmodern feminism, Islamic feminism, Jewish feminism, Christian feminism and post-structural feminism.

Feminism is a bedrock in Women's Studies and or Gender Studies within academia, but it is also a specialty area within other academic disciplines like Education, the Humanities, Fine Arts, Health Sciences and within all the Social Sciences, including Anthropology, Linguistics, Communications and Psychology. Some feminist scholars explore gendered ways of speaking, learning, thinking, writing, creating, performing and counseling as well as investigate gender-specific health or medical concerns, family and domestic realities, and legal rights and access to representation. There are also those focused on the rewriting of history to include women as well as those searching out new female stories and novel ways to write them. Some examine literary theory and the way women and women's lives are seen in literature and art, as well as the ways women have used literature and language to shed light on their experiences as women. There are a multitude of ways feminism intersects with a host of academic discussions.

Because of the various strands and understandings of feminism, the word is extremely difficult to define. It is better to refer to it as plural: *feminisms*. We can only try to pick out some common characteristics of the varieties of feminism. Most are, at least sometimes, critiques of *patriarchy* (the hierarchy of the male) or critiques of *misogyny* (the hatred of the female). It may be safe to say that all feminisms are a disenchantment of some sort with an *androcentric* society, one which sees the male experience as the central point of reference of 'the norm', while the female experience is what is 'marked', what is different, what is not 'norm' and what is seen as 'other'.

There are many examples of how patriarchy is revealed in language use. For example, the word 'waiter' is perceived as the 'norm' or the 'unmarked' word used in our everyday language, while 'waitress' is the marked variation – it is a change from the 'norm'. The use of the word 'waitress' highlights the server as different from a waiter; this is what is meant by 'marked'. In educational theory, Swiss theorist, Jean Piaget, based his theory of social development on boys thus privileging the male experience as the 'norm', or, that which is presented and understood as universal: there were no girls in Piaget's research. Feminisms are concerned with the ways these kinds of assumptions in society exist and search for ways they can be interrupted and interrogated for the sake of those born – or who identify as – female. Feminisms explore the effects of assumed privilege, examine and expose these outcomes in a quest for reasonable accountability, and pursue basic social justice and human rights. Feminisms seek out which voices and stories get heard in society and which do not, including in the realms of politics, academia, classrooms, churches and families. Feminisms concern themselves with the perceived inferiority of women and the discrimination women encounter because of their sex and because of assumptions about femininity itself, while some women themselves collude in the perpetuation of these attitudes.

Especially in the latter half of the 20th century, feminisms have also been characterized by major American movements like the *Equal Rights Amendment* and the *National Organization of Women*. These mid-century American incarnations of feminisms (and other similar efforts in the United Kingdom, Canada, Australia and around the world) insisted that women be free to pursue careers and economic independence as well as to have freedom from any male-based oppression in their personal or workplace relationships. This particular wave of feminism in the West (the second wave) followed closely on the heels of the 1950s post-war era, a decade with a heavy domestic emphasis. The 1960s and 1970s was a uniquely potent period for the realignment of established attitudes, including (but not limited to) those surrounding gender roles. Indeed, the period hosted a plethora of anti-establishment movements. The entire era in the United States was framed by the anti-Vietnam war protests and the fight for Civil Rights. Feminism as experienced in the 1960s was inspired by *consciousness raising groups* where women gathered together to question and reject their restrictive role in society. These *baby-boomers* (those born between 1945 and 1964) propelled an unprecedented revolution regarding social roles, politics, religion, affluence, philosophy and the politics of war and peace. Challenging sex/gender roles was a part of these other societal shifts. The 1960s and its *sexual revolution* challenged the traditional models of male-female relationships.

By the 1970s and 1980s, Western societies saw many resulting legal reforms, such as equal pay for equal work, more accessible divorce laws, more legal access to abortion, increased day care options, and more affirmative action in both the workplace and in educational opportunities. Quite rightly, many societies have a lot to thank second wave feminism for in regards to the improvement in much of women's freedom – particularly in the West. The issue of women and their lives on the margins of power entered the social consciousness and changed enormously in the workforce, in university programs, in the literary canon and in family dynamics.

Importantly, the notion of feminism itself must be understood as much, much older than the second wave incarnation; the study of and concern for women and women's experiences reaches much further back. Major early feminist thinkers include England's Mary Wollstonecraft who, as an extension of the Enlightenment movement in general, wrote *A Vindication of the Rights of Woman* in 1792. Wollstonecraft criticized the lack of rigorous education for girls in 18th-century England as related to their weaker positions in society. She believed that women couldn't possibly hold positions of power if they lacked the training to do so. She saw it as imperative that society educate its women. American Sarah Moore Grimké wrote *Letters on the Equality of the Sexes* in the early 1800s. In 1843, Sojourner Truth gave her 'Ain't I a Woman?' speech as part of the emerging feminist movement in and around New York State. American suffragist Elizabeth Cady Stanton wrote *The Woman's Bible* in 1895, a document offering a woman's perspective on Biblical events. There were also various writers from the Women's Christian Temperance Movement who established the YWCA and influenced major prison reforms throughout the British Empire, including Australia, New Zealand and Canada, among many other nations around the world. Britain's Emmeline Pankhurst and her universal suffrage movement promoted the vote for British women. The Suffrage movement took at least 50 years to successfully secure voting rights for women; this movement is known as 'the first wave'. In many ways, this wave also includes those who focused on women's service and experience in the two world wars and between the wars, such as the flappers in the jazz age and the Depression Era reforms led by American Eleanor Roosevelt. England's Virginia Woolf's feminist lectures to the University of Cambridge's Girton Ladies College, compiled in *A Room of One's Own*, was published in 1928. France's Simone de Beauvoir wrote *The Second Sex* in 1949. Both of these texts became foundational to later efforts to promote equality among the sexes.

All these women and a host of others were established as major world writers, thinkers and politicians long before 1960s feminists such as Betty Friedan and Gloria Steinem championed feminism for white, upper middle class, suburban American women. The second wave centered itself in many ways on the boredom such women were experiencing. Allison Pease (2012) addresses this phenomenon as 'the culture of boredom', in which the search for meaning became a central premise. This 'practice of self-reflection' created desire but with no clear object or objective. There is a lingering view of feminism as both political and militant. This opinion is a direct result of the perception of how the feminists of the 1960s advocated for equality. This perceived militancy has detracted many potential feminists (i.e. anyone who believes in the innate equality of women and men) from encountering the more robust literature that highlights how critical feminism has been around the world. Feminism continues to debate significant issues unique to (or almost always uniquely centered on) women: rape, domestic violence, pornography, prostitution, female circumcision, self-harm, dowry crimes, or women's rights to education or legal protection. Anyone connected to academia today recognizes the basic gifts of feminist thought to our daily lives.

The patriarchal system entrenched in Western society can be seen in the work of early 20th century thinkers, such as Otto Jespersen (1922). He suggested that women spoke in ways different from men because they were simply unable to speak in strong, coherent sentences or with an extensive vocabulary. He believed that the greatest orators of history were men because of innate abilities in them that were rarely found in women. This was the prevalent view at the time. However, it was not the only view. There were many individuals who suggested various reasons for the perceived discrepancies between the ways in which women and men wrote and spoke. Virginia Woolf (1928), in *A Room of One's Own*, suggested that women's absence from positions of power had to do with the lack of opportunity for women to assume those positions and not with an innate weakness in those born female. In other words, women were not innately unable to be innovative or sophisticated in thought or language; however, they lacked the educational and economic opportunities that were available to men.

Sex and Gender

Important to mention is what *gender* is understood to be and how it is distinct from *sex*. For most people, our sex is determined by being born male or female. However, our gender refers to the ways in which masculinity and femininity are enacted; gender is a social construct, a set of behaviors, related to our sex but quite distinct from it. Our sex affects how we interact with the world because of what is linked to it (for example, the capacity to give birth) and what is associated with the linking of 'maleness' and 'female-ness' to those around us. Sex is, therefore, related to gender but it is not the same thing. The current debates surrounding one's sexual identity as distinct from one's biological sex are centered around this very reality. Gender is a social category of behavior and is not an innate feature. It is, however, strongly associated with the social divisions made on the basis of sex. Meanwhile, language plays a major role in establishing and sustaining these divisions. Though the word 'gender' is also a grammatical category in some languages (such as the 'masculine' or 'feminine' used for syntactic meaning in such languages as French), the social sciences use the concept of gender as a social category. 'Masculine' and 'feminine' are understood as behavioral categories usually – but not necessarily – ascribed to and aligned with those born with the correlative sex. Those born male are associated with, or per-haps are compelled to embody, behaviors that are perceived and under-stood as masculine, while those born female are associated with, or are compelled to embody, behaviors that are perceived and understood by society as feminine.

This critical distinction between *sex* and *gender* was first articulated by a British feminist in the early 1970s. Anne Oakley (1972) defined sex as biologi-cally based, a matter of physiology, something related to genes, gonads, hor-mones and anatomy. The female ova contain the female sex chromosome X; a male sperm contains either X or Y chromosomes. Sex has been understood as essentially binary: one is *either* male *or* female. Today's discussions of transgenderism challenge these traditional understandings yet, for the majority of people, the sex one is born with is fixed.

Gender, then, is *socially constructed*: it is something learned from the environments that surround us. Social scientists believe that we acquire characteristics and behaviors because of how they are understood by the people or communities in our lives: we gradually become more or less mas-culine or more or less feminine based on the responses of those to whom we belong. We behave in certain gendered ways in various circumstances for a variety of reasons, especially in regards to our sense of who we are – our personal identities and agency. *Agency* refers to one's capacity to originate and direct one's own actions in response to the prevailing environment. It involves a sense of control, power and awareness of one's self. Whether consciously or not, we enact who we are based largely on how others construct us – but, we also represent ourselves on our own sense of agency.

Gender is certainly not binary; one is not masculine *or* feminine, but is rather a combination of many characteristics that could be understood as either or both depending on the context and relationship. The fact that we align certain behaviors or attitudes as masculine or feminine reveals how society affects our view of the world. We can say someone is 'more masculine' or 'more feminine' – for example, we can say someone is 'very manly' or 'a girlie girl'. Grammatically, as well as physiologically, we cannot say one is *maler*. We perform gender roles found on a continuum of masculine and feminine characteristics; this is why we can say that we are *gendered* and are involved in the process of our own gendering throughout our lives.

The process of 'doing gender' is something that begins before birth: many new parents know the sex of their baby months before the birth and, thus, begin to associate certain gender characteristics with their unborn baby. They buy pink clothes for baby girls and blue clothes for baby boys. They imagine particular future experiences because of their baby's sex. Throughout infancy, early childhood, the school years, adolescence, early adulthood, even into middle age and as seniors, we are responded to based on our gender performance and, at some level, we respond to others in the same way. In other words, we are gendered. If gender was exclusively a matter of one's biological sex, then we would see the same displays of gender roles, behaviors and attitudes across all cultures, across all time periods, and across all age groups; but we do not. There is extraordinary diversity. The way my mother performed her gender as a young woman in the 1950s is quite different from the way I behaved, felt and spoke as a young woman in the 1980s, and this performance of gender is different yet again from my daughter's genderedness as a young woman in the 21st century. We have different tastes, expectations, values, behaviors and life experiences that are linked to the gender worlds of our particular place and time. Also, a woman of my similar age but living in a dramatically different culture (say, in the Congo) has a different set of life experiences from me that may cause her to enact her feminine gender in a completely different way. It is important, then, to understand that gender performances are not universal, but that gender as a social construct is a universal ingredient influencing the way we live our lives and understand each other in our partic-ular circumstances.

Deborah Cameron (2008) characterizes a 'pluralizing' of masculinities and femininities as seeing the many different ways language is 'deployed' in various settings to produce a whole plethora of masculinities and feminini-ties. In this way, we inhabit and engender social contexts. Some of our notions of gender are often more strongly related to stage of life rather than one's sex. For example, women are viewed as nurturing but mainly in con-nection with motherhood and not necessarily during a woman's teen years or in old age. Generalizations about women and men simply cannot be maintained given the considerable variation that exists across gender groups at intersections with one's social class, ethnicity, race and context over one's lifetime.

Arguably, the most significant theoretic work to influence the field of language and gender has been Judith Butler's (1990) *Gender Trouble* in which she articulates her notion of 'performativity'; she sees gender as something we do, not something we are. According to Butler, gender is not fixed – and it is not even very stable. In this view, we are not governed by a certain 'essence' of an individual; rather gender '*emerges* in discourse and in other *semiotic* practices' (Ehrlich & Meyerhoff, 2014: 4). As individuals, we do not act out of a pre-existing gender; instead we are involved with others in 'doing' gender. In so many ways we are rehearsed into our gender roles, like being prepared for a part in a play. Over our whole lives and particularly in our early formative years, we are conditioned, prompted and prodded to behave in acceptable ways so that our gender (and our community's under-standing of it) aligns with our sex.

Not all scholars agree fully with Butler's ideas about performativity. Instead, and often for political engagement, a 'strategic essentialism' (groups working together as a unit) can be critical in addressing social issues like rac-ism, systemic sexism and other social divisions. Placing the entire human experience on the individual takes away focus from systemic injustices where marginalized groups can affect any change. In fact, feminism itself is based on this very idea: women, and men who care about the lives of women, need to work together to create a more just world.

The tricky part is the extent to which behaviors are biologically deter-mined and which behaviors are learned through social experiences. Which behaviors exist because of one's gender identity? Which ones are based in physiology? Some gender and sex roles are fairly straightforward; for exam-ple, since women bear children, they are in a special position to be mothers and be motherly. And yet, nurturing behaviors are not sex-based: either a man or a woman can similarly soothe a crying child.

There is also evidence suggesting that some men tend to be more aggressive than some women; for example, more men are convicted of violent crime. But is aggression related to biology – to the higher levels of testosterone in those born male, for example – or is it related to the way boys are handled and viewed by society so that over time they become more aggressive? Perhaps it is both. One wonders why young boys, whose testosterone levels are the same as young girls in early childhood, demonstrate a tendency towards aggression even then? Perhaps some little boys are more aggressive than some little girls because of how society interprets their actions as aggressive and, thereby, inadvertently develops them as aggressive. For example, we give boys toy guns and other tools that encourage aggressive behavior. The tendency for aggression may be a sex-based biological characteristic, but it also may be an aspect of gender (masculinity) – something socially constructed, socially valued and socially located. Recent advancements in our understanding of this interplay have been possible because of growing scientific research that has enhanced our understanding of the interplay between sex and gender through new advances in brain imaging and new explanations of how environment is a key factor in gendering children.

Increasing research on the brain has allowed us some deeper awareness about gender. There is absolutely no way we can see 'gender' in a brain any more than we can see race, ethnicity or social class. Only age is visible in an image of a brain. That said, the brain develops various aspects as we grow older; the brain synapses are formed after birth so that what is environmental (i.e. gender) can appear to be biologically based. Our brain chemistry is altered by the circumstances in which we live. We can see the effects of poverty on brain development, for instance. In a similar way, we can see the effects of gender in altering brain development so that it's trickier to make a nature/nurture argument when nurture itself becomes nature. That is, social construction influences brain development itself.

Mary Talbot's (1998) work cautioned against simply mapping gender onto sex. Mapping gender onto sex comes with an assumption or belief that 'socially determined differences between women and men are natural and inevitable' (p. 9). Also, viewing sex and gender as the same thing connects to the promotion of rigid gender roles and to the justifications for white, male privilege and power. Such thinking is known as *biological determinism*. With this view, we can say things like 'women are like that' and thus dismiss something more complex about being human and understanding human experience as something infinitely more mysterious and complicated. If the distinction between sex and gender is blurred or completely erased so that 'sex' is the same as 'gender', then certain restrictions and demands can be placed on both sexes. In the case of women, the phrase 'women are like that' becomes, even more problematically, 'women are only like that' or 'women must be like that'.

Biological determinism is also referred to as *essentialism*. This perspective tries to establish and affirm a genetic or 'essential' basis for our behaviors and life trajectories. Racial views also fall victim to this kind of thinking, like believing that all Black people are musical because it's 'in their blood'. Obviously, this is a *stereotype*; some Black people are musical but not all. It is also worth considering that some feminists themselves hold to essentialism, such as Andrea Dworkin (1981) who said, 'violence is male and the male is the penis' (p. 515). To her, the essence of a male person is to be violent. To some, it is 'in their blood' to commit certain crimes (like rape) or to imagine their power when viewing pornography. More men do commit rape and look at pornography, but this does not and cannot imply that *all* men would do so simply on account of their having a penis. This line of thinking is limited because it destroys our ability to create meaningful and authentic lives and to see people in their own right as people first. Biology plays a major part in forming our life experiences, but the ways we are responded to throughout our lives and the ways we are socially constructed by those around us is also very influential.

I think it is helpful to hold a 'both/and' view of gender and sex, gender identity, and sexual identity, rather than an 'either/or' view. Those who see the human experience as a complex mystery cannot limit people based on their sex or gender or race or other sociological variables. Why? Because an understanding of such variables helps locate us as part of a group while also being distinct and unique persons.

For any claim by biological determinists (e.g. 'women are better at languages'), there is a challenging counterclaim (e.g. 'men are better public speakers'). Some scholars suggested in the early 1990s that 'studies of difference' ultimately have a political dimension. Why do we want to find differences? Whose purposes are being served if we see differences? Deborah Cameron (1992) points out that one's understanding of gender often aligns with larger political or philosophical views.

LGBTQ+ Terminology

The rise of LGBTQ+ cultures has become a central aspect of Women's and Gender Studies research. LGBTQ stands for lesbian, gay, bisexual, transgender and queer or questioning, with an added plus sign (+) to indicate other sexual identities. In use since the 1990s, the term is an adaptation of the earlier form, LGB. American activists in the mid-1980s felt that the term 'gay community' did not accurately represent all those to whom it referred. Today, in most English-speaking countries, the term LGBTQ+ is intended to emphasize the diversity of sexualities and gender identities.

Since the mid-1990s, the addition of Q has embraced those who identify as *Queer* or who are *Questioning* their sexuality. Transgender (or simply 'trans') is a term used to describe those whose gender identity and/or gender expression (how they outwardly demonstrate their gender) differs from the sex they were born with and who may seek to 'transition' their bodies to the sex which better matches their gender identities. Sometimes the addition of I is also added to include those who identify as *intersex*. Hence, the acronym LGBTIQ or LGBTQI is also gaining acceptance, among other variations, though LGBTQ+ seems to be the more common term.

All that said, K.M. Harris's (2013) online survey revealed that most people who identify with the LGBTQ community do so because of Q: most are questioning their sexuality, which may reflect the great uncertainty and external pressures surrounding sexuality itself. Queer Studies explores the related realities concerning sexuality; it is viewed as a subsection of Gender Studies and is an emerging research field of its own as an extension of 'critical identities' that embrace post-colonial ideals of dismantling patriarchy.

The terminology itself, which has led to the variety of aforementioned acronyms, has also changed over time. 'Third Gender' was the term in the middle of the 19th century. 'Homosexual' and 'homophile' were commonly used in the 1950s and 1960s. By the 1970s, 'gay' was common and was the preferred word of the community itself. 'Sexual minority' was also used at the time. The evolving terminology highlights the development of the community as well as signals certain areas of dispute. Each group within the LGBTQ+ categories have had to assert their inclusion, while others have felt that adding more letters diminishes the goals of their particular group. For example, some gays and lesbians are less accepting than one might expect of transgender people who identify as straight, saying that they are acting out gender stereotypes and/or are simply afraid to come out.

In any case, the term LGBT is widely accepted in the West and is viewed as a positive symbol of inclusion. The order of the letters can be viewed as a nod to feminism (starting with the letter L for Lesbian). Other variants like 'pansexual' or 'omnisexual' are viewed as part of the B category: bisexuality. Likewise, 'intersex' falls into the category of transgender, while the National LGBTI Health Alliance recognizes 'intersex' as a biological attribute distinct from gender identity and sexual orientation. *Cisgendered* and *non-cisgendered* are terms gaining in popularity. Of note, the term SLG (same-loving gender) is sometimes used in the African-American community which sees LGBT as distinctly concerned with the White community.

Regardless of the letters used (and there are a host of possibilities), not all people associated with gay or lesbian or the other categories approve of the jargon, citing it as existing for political and social solidarity that normally aligns with gay pride marches or events. Not all LGBT people support LGBT activism nor are they a part of such efforts, viewing the term as based on LGBT stereotypes and suppressing of the individuality of LGBT people. On the BBC website, journalist Julie Bindel (2014) questioned the bracketing together of LGBTQ+ people as though they all 'share the same issues, values, and goals'. Other useful terminology includes:

Mx: gender-neutral title (rather than Mr, Ms, etc.)

Pansexual/Omnisexual: someone attracted to all members of all gender identities/expressions

Skoliosexual: a person attracted to people who are *non-cisgender* (i.e. transgender)

Ze/Hir: alternate, gender-neutral pronouns preferred by some trans people

(*Esquire* Magazine, 2016: 146–147)

One of the most recent changes to the English language is the growing use of the pronoun 'they' as a singular pronoun referring to either a woman or man. It has also recently been used by transgender people to avoid 'he' or 'she' when they are referred to. 'They' is seen as a better fit with ambiguous sex/gender identities. The word 'they' was recognized in 2015 as the 'Word of the Year' by the American Dialect Society, yet these discussions go back 40 years at least (Bodine, 1975). The increasing use of the gender-neutral pronoun 'ze' is also connected to the concern with and power of language to define who we are.

Neoliberalism, the New Feminism and Globalization

Neoliberalism is a term first used in the 1930s in regards to economic policy related to deregulation. It was first identified as a concept in reference to 19th-century ideas concerning 'laissez faire' economics where transactions between people could be free from any governmental involvement. A hundred years later, in the 1980s, this meant supporting *economic liberalization*, including privatization, deregulation, free trade, reductions in government spending to increase the role of the private sector in the economy or, rather, the role of government in the private sector. Neoliberalism is associated with policies introduced by Margaret Thatcher in Britain and Ronald Reagan in the United States. Some economists and academics point to these leaders' policies as the root of the financial crisis of 2008 (World Health Organization, online). Since the 1980s, the term has been used by a whole range of scholars in various social sciences as well as employed in relation to the attitudes and effects of neoliberalism on a range of contexts.

The impact of the 2008 global economic crisis was a prime example of neoliberal economics. As such, some new scholarship has criticized neoliberalism as being unjust and abusive in so far as it pits the poor against the wealthy. An important critique involves social class. According to critics of neoliberalism, not all members of any society have equal access to the law or to information. This is because access to information is not free, or not freely available. This ignorance has associated costs. The neoliberal ideas concerning the power of the individual have been to the advantage of capitalist elites who can use their wealth as personal markers of success ('we worked for our wealth'); in this scenario, the wealthy argue that the poor are equally able to achieve these same levels of wealth if they so desire. The working poor, then, are viewed as responsible for their own individual failure to gain wealth. In a neoliberal society, capitalism has allowed capitalists free range in making money without concerns for any social assistance programs. If the poor are entirely responsible for their poverty, why would social assistance of any kind be needed? If one believes that all people create their own circumstances, then those with more can keep amassing wealth without any impetus to help others who struggle.

Feminists have aggressively criticized neoliberalism for its negative effect on those who are disenfranchised, including those in the female workforce across the world, especially in the global south. Feminists see neoliberalism as benefitting masculinist objectives to dominate economic and geopolitical thinking. Women's experiences in non-industrialized countries have, in many ways, been disastrous because of modernist/neoliberal claims that development benefits everyone when this is clearly untrue: cheaper labor in developing countries enhances profits for the wealthy in the West. They do not benefit from the generated riches. Feminists say that participation in the economy does not further equality in gender relations. For example, Peterson (2015) says, 'Employers in the global south have perceptions about feminine labor and seek workers who are perceived to be undemanding, docile, and willing to accept low wages' (p. 180). As such, the exploitation of female workers is very widespread and is a prevailing concern in feminist social critique. When economic conditions deteriorate, women are culturally expected to fill in the gap in spite of few resources.

'Post-Feminism' relates to neoliberalism. It is a shift away from a collective movement towards a conviction that individual women are solely responsible for their own successes or failures. It empties liberal feminism of its moral compass, moving feminism as a structural force and group to an individual's problem to solve for themselves. The neoliberal shift within feminism neutralizes any collective uprising and transfers concern for women's equality from the public to the individual. This is post-feminism. This is a sad development, in my opinion, because it undermines feminism's key goal of changing unjust social conditions for all women. Instead, post-feminism is an individual journey of discovery, placing responsibility for failure or injustice totally in the hands of the woman herself. Catherine Rottenberg (2014) provides a helpful explanation: 'Shifting away from the power and possibilities of the collective means feminism is without its analyses of the structures of male/masculinist "dominance, power and privilege"' (p. 424). This is a troubling trend indeed, which seems to have grown considerably in the last 10 years. In neoliberalism, the 'feminist subject' accepts 'full responsibility for her own well-being and self-care' (2014: 424).

Post-feminism doesn't negate the existence of or need for feminists. Today's generation of feminists are often referred to as 'new feminists'. New feminism comes with a greater understanding of geopolitical realities than the second wave feminists could have foreseen. Can feminisms tackle neoliberalism (a major force in the world's economy and social order) and its relationship with globalization? The ways forward are difficult to predict. For this very reason, feminism has become increasingly relevant (not less) in understanding shifting world powers and alliances.

Catherine Redfern and Kristen Aune (2013) in their book, *Reclaiming the F Word: Feminism Today*, articulate the rising hopes and efforts of the new generation. They point out that 75% of feminists today are under the age of 35. These new activists are confident that the relevance of feminism today is as great as ever. They declare that new feminisms are 'liberating, diverse, challenging, exciting, relevant and inclusive [...]. In an increasingly global society, feminism transcends national boundaries' (p. x). New feminisms are emerging to deal with the problems associated with neoliberalism and globalization, and they see gender relations as a continuing and central concern the world over. Where educational opportunities for girls in the West have flourished, much is needed for girls in developing nations. Where women in western cultures have, at least practically speaking, freedom of mobility and safe ways out of abusive marriages, women in developing countries do not and so desperately need the global sisterhood to help bring more personal freedom to their lives. An understanding of feminism in opposition to neoliberalism is also necessary for those new to the field: feminists work together to enhance the experiences of women (and, relatedly, men) throughout the world. An individualist focus does not a civil and just society make.

Summing Up

- Feminism is the policy, practice or advocacy of political, economic and social equality for women. It has a long history and a complicated relationship with contemporary society.
- Our sex is usually determined by our being born male or female, while gender is the complex and fluid social category of behaviors often (but not necessarily) associated with our biological sex.
- Terminology needed to best represent the attention now paid to people who are **non-cisgendered** is important; it reveals the realities, situations and concerns of a variety of people.
- Neoliberal ideas have made life less equitable (not more) because it provides advantages to those already benefiting from capitalism. The rise of individualism has caused less concern for structural inequalities and unbridled concern for the self over others.

2

Language as Gendered

. . . .

Clearly she was expected to say something,
but panic at having to speak stole the thoughts from her head.

Shannon Hale, *The Goose Girl*

Language is often considered to be a neutral and passive phenomenon whose main function is to communicate or reflect whatever is happening in society. Nevertheless, language is not value free; language can be a source for good or a tool of oppression. It is not just a reflection of society, but is involved in the construction and perpetuation of social realities. This chapter explores key ways language use can reveal and create gender identities.

Grappling with the wide variety of ways that language *reflects* society's attitudes concerning gender is vital to understanding gender and language. Equally crucial is working to understand how language *constructs* attitudes towards gender roles and expectations. Consider the way women are sometimes addressed in public discourse as 'girl' (i.e. 'We have a new *girl* at the office') whereas men are rarely referred to as 'boy' in a similar context. This reality reveals a patriarchal society that benefits in some way by referring to a grown, professional woman as a child. The sentence perpetuates this attitude. The attitude can be spotted in various situations and circumstances where language can be seen to reveal gendered lives as well as to reinforce performances of gender in what, how and why we say the things we do.

Early in the 20th century, Edward Sapir (1929) and his graduate student, Benjamin Whorf, American linguists and anthropologists, proclaimed that 'the limits of one's language are the limits of one's world'. This sentiment, known as the *Sapir–Whorf Hypothesis*, sees a systemic relationship between one's language and how one understands the world around oneself (Sapir, 1929). This hypothesis suggested that language can only reflect our lived experiences and shape our experiences. Current researchers are more critical of this stance because of the very real possibility that we have the ability to experience things that we cannot yet articulate. Even if we don't have a word, expression or way of expressing a certain notion or feeling, this does not mean we do not experience it. For example, a woman in the 19th century might well have experienced 'domestic abuse' well before such a term existed. This means the term reflected the reality rather than creating it. In so many ways language aligns with creativity and idiosyncratic possibilities – language use is highly artistic, imaginative and fluid throughout time and in various communities. In the example of a woman being referred to as a 'girl', perhaps the use of the term 'girl' displays an ironic and sophisticated understanding of power relations rather than serving as evidence of society's dismissive views of what is female. Understanding context, intentions and motivations are critical in understanding gender and language. It is within these complexities that the relationship between language and gender emerges.

We can and do use language to change attitudes and develop society and, thus, we do change our private understandings of our own realities with the development of new words, phrases, diction, etc. Thinking about language and gender is related to the feminist concerns of stopping any continued systematic inequalities that exist between men and women. This does not equate with an arbitrary political goal, but to human rights. Even for those who see differences between women and men with regards to roles of leadership can't deny that language is a key tool that can and is used to create a certain understanding of things. Language plays a complex part in reflecting, creating and sustaining our own genderedness and the genderedness of others. The study of language plays a big part in changing gendered divisions precisely because it reveals them. In this regard, it is worth considering the previous and residual view in society of the feminine as deficient and the masculine as powerful as a way to move towards some alternative, more equitable understandings.

Sexism as a term was first coined in the 1960s, along with the term *racism*, to describe discrimination in society based on certain permanent personal traits, including being born female or male or being born black or white. Sexism helps identify the historical patriarchal hierarchy that has existed, and in many ways throughout the world continues to exist, between men and women where one (the man) is considered *the norm* and the other (the woman) is marked as *the other*. In this view, *the other* can be exploited, manipulated, or constrained by the norm because of the difference from what is considered the usual experience. In Gender Studies, this *othering* is usually associated with women; however, othering can also be based on race, religion, sexual orientation, disabilities or any trait or condition that is viewed as different from what is viewed as 'normal' in any given society or community.

The questions and criticisms of sexist language have emerged because of a concern that language is a powerful medium through which the world functions. One example of *gender bias* seen in language use is the case of pronouns, particularly the generic use of 'he' or 'him' to refer to both men and women. Feminist linguists, such as Dale Spender in the early 1980s, believed that language had been historically 'man-made', and that was why the male forms are viewed as what is normal – because they reflect the male's legitimate position in society, while female forms are 'deviant'. Some have claimed that the use of generics (such as 'mankind' to refer to both men and women) reinforces this binary that sees the male and masculine as the norm and the female and feminine as the 'not norm'. Feminists also objected to the use of generic expressions because of what cannot be truly generic. We might be able to say, 'Man is a lonely creature' to imply all people, but we cannot say, 'Man has difficulty in childbirth' for the obvious reason that individuals born biologically male cannot give birth. Graddol and Swann (1989) wrote extensively on such sexist language in the 1980s and 1990s and considered such claims as expressions that limit an understanding of the human experience. Examples such as 'woman doctor' or 'male nurse' and the connotations of certain seemingly neutral terms, such as 'lady' or 'bachelor', or even 'girl' or 'mothering', need our reflection and care because they reflect our understanding of what is *normative* concerning gendered expectations.

Generic expressions are also understood to have prevented women from expressing and raising consciousness about their own experiences as legitimately human – preventing women from speaking with their own *voice* (Gilligan, 1982). Their invisibility in certain situations, and associated silence, has been seen as perpetuating gender assumptions in society to the extent that we have come to see what is male and experienced by males as the point of reference for everybody.

Sexist language reveals stereotypes of females and males, sometimes to the disadvantage of males, but more often to the disadvantage of females. This sexism in language is not exclusive to English, though it is very much present there. Robin Lakoff (1975) used the example of 'master' versus 'mistress' to make the point that there are unequal connotations which surround these terms – and certainly to the detriment of those born female. The word 'master' has strong and powerful connotations, while 'mistress' has come to mean a woman of questionable legitimacy or a temptress.

Sexist language also results in the depiction of women as passive objects rather than active subjects on the basis of their appearance ('a blonde') or on the basis of their domestic roles ('a mother of two') when similar depictions in similar contexts would not be made of men. These depictions of women trivialize them and, by placing them in the passive object position, put an extra level of judgment on them for being less vital in society than men. Men can be trivialized and negatively judged by sexist language as well ('what a stud') but feminists contend that the connotations in such examples are not as severe or limiting in the same way as they are for women; indeed, viewing a man as an object of desire may be understood by both men and women as flirtatious and affirming, but our society's patriarchal history means that gendered connotations are not the same.

Ultimately, feminist linguists hope that attention to language use can denaturalize an assumed male privilege and the patriarchal system that secures it, believing that this will loosen gender roles for both males and females. But sexist language is not only located in the content or meanings of specific words or phrases. It is also found in dialogue, in discourse, and in the meanings and communication created by speech styles or patterns in longer spoken texts and within conversations. Language changes from one context to another, from one community to another, and from one time period to another. Language changes as a result of social, political and economic processes. It changes because of modifications to lifestyle, or because of encounters with technologies, media and migration. Language also changes as a result of the dynamic relationship between conservation and innovation. As such, an awareness of sexist language can prompt new ways of speaking about the human experience. Ultimately, our own language use can reveal our awareness or our lack of awareness of human complexity.

Studies on the nature of language that were done throughout the 1960s and 1970s attempted to understand demographic groups, ultimately making claims such as that men speak more vernacularly (casually) than women do. The best known work of this type was done by William Labov, in New York (1966). Of note in his work was the notion of linguistic change. The possibility that language is stylistic and based on sex led Labov and other scholars to suggest that men are more at ease in social settings and that women are more anxious and in need of achieving a certain level of respectability. Women, therefore, would speak in more correct ways because using standard language is an important access to legitimacy. Men, alternatively, can be and are more creative with language since they are unmarked, the norm and legitimate. This line of research is over 50 years old. Nevertheless, the study of language use in social relationships still finds these gendered tendencies/variations of men and women in certain circumstances.

Over 40 years ago, Peter Trudgill (1974) conducted a survey in Norwich, England, modeled on Labov's New York study. He, too, attempted to establish the variation of formality that occurs in various settings and often along gender lines. However, Trudgill found that women claimed to use more standard speech than they actually did while men claimed to use more vernacular speech than was truly present in their words spoken. In response, Trudgill suggested that sex-exclusive kinds of differences are a result of social attitudes about the 'proper' or 'acceptable' speech of women and men while not based on actual speech patterns at all. That is, women are thought to be more status-conscious than men and, therefore, we see them as more aware of the significance of linguistic variables. But why would we do this? Possible explanations include society's view of women's social position as one that is less secure: we believe that women need to secure and signal their social status, and that they must use language as a way to do this. This possibility is at the core of Sheryl Sandberg's (2015) very popular ideas found in her celebrated bestseller, *Lean In: Women, Work and the Will to Lead*. She says that speaking in powerful ways can make someone powerful. Or, if someone speaks with more reticence, people come to view this person as less significant. Men in western society are often rated by their occupation or their earning power, and so we perceive their use of language as more necessary and authoritative. If they are not successful in such ways, their use of language will reveal that as well, and our perceptions of their speech will also align with our views that they lack authority or legitimacy.

Language and Power

Gendered language debates in previous decades were guided by two main theoretical positions: *the theory of deficit or dominance* (popular in the 1970s through the 1980s) and *the theory of difference* (popular in the 1990s). The first position saw any sex/gender differences found in language use as a result of women being dominated by men in various interactions across time and space. The second position viewed women and men as belonging to distinct sub-cultures that were simply and benignly different – no one was being dominated and no one was doing the dominating. Both of these 20th-century views reflected the political climate at particular times. The 21st century, however, has seen the study of gender move well beyond these two views. Today's rich research environment expands earlier analyses by taking into account contexts and situations that position gender and language performances as always 'located' somewhere and somehow. This newer understanding allows for a wide variety of circumstances to be considered across the world and across cultural divides.

Back in 1975, Robin Lakoff published her account of what made up 'women's language'. She put forward a set of basic assumptions about how women speak. These features were only representative of her own local community of upper-class white women in 1970s New York since it was this context that provided all the data. Despite the limited population from which she drew her conclusions, she seemed to be making claims about 'women' as a global category. Today's new feminists would find her method deeply flawed in so far as they would see circumstances as much more central to language choices than Lakoff's study allowed. Her publication was seminal to the field. She claimed that women used:

- *Hedges*, such as 'sort of', 'kind of', 'it seems like'
- *(super)polite forms*, like 'Would you mind...', 'I'd appreciate it if...', '...if you don't mind'
- *tag questions*, like 'You're going to dinner, aren't you?'
- *italics* and intonational emphasis equal to underlining words, like 'so', 'very', 'quite'
- *empty adjectives*, such as 'divine', 'lovely' and 'adorable'
- *hypercorrect grammar and pronunciation*; women used precise prestige grammar and clear enunciation
- *more back-channel support*, such as nodding one's head or offering indications when listening to encourage the speaker to continue
- *a special lexicon*; women used more words for things such as colors
- *question intonation in declarative statements*; women made declarative statements into questions by raising the pitch of their voice at the end of a statement, expressing uncertainty
- *avoidance of coarse language or expletives*
- *indirect commands and requests*, such as 'My, isn't it cold in here?' as a request to turn the heat on or close a window
- *more intensifiers*, especially 'so' and 'very' (e.g. 'I am *so* glad you came!')

(adapted from Lakoff, 1975: 53–55)

Other tendencies emerged, such as women also spoke with direct quotations while men paraphrased more often. They used 'wh-' imperatives, such as

'Why don't you open the door?'. They spoke less frequently. They overused qualifiers; for example, 'I think that...'. They offered more apologies for no particular reason; for instance, 'I'm sorry, but I think that...'. Modal constructions, such as 'can', 'would', 'should', 'ought' (e.g. 'Should we turn up the heat?') were also considered part of feminine speech style. Moreover, women lacked a sense of humour, and they would stop speaking when interrupted while men would not.

Lakoff claimed that the linguistic features that she noted were typical of women's speech indicated insecurity on the part of many women. She wrote:

> Women's speech seems in general to contain more instances of 'well', 'you know', 'kind of', and so forth: words that convey the sense that the speaker is uncertain about what [she] is saying. (p. 53)

It is from this view that claims can be made about changing language patterns deliberately to become more powerful in the workplace or in positions of leadership. More recent additions to the sense of female language is the use of 'vocal fry', known as 'the speaking style afflicting American women or the verbal tic of doom'. It is the latest 'uptalk' or 'valleyspeak' of the 'ditzy girl' – an artificial dumbing down of the sound of one's language use in order to be seen as less than or smaller than people with more power (men, presumably) or could also signal confidence in the speaker, depending on context.[1] Vocal fry describes a specific sound quality caused by movements in the vocal folds. It's also known as creaky voice or as 'the way a Kardashian speaks'.[2] As with all performances of gender, language use reveals attitudes and basic worldviews; the vocal fry says something about one's attitude and the belonging to a certain group.

Lakoff believed that women qualified their statements in many ways because of their uncertainty and because they wanted to be (or at least felt most comfortable being) subordinate to others so as not to overwhelm or overstep their place. Lakoff's ideas sparked other interpretations of women's language patterns or tendencies, however. British academic Deborah Cameron (1998) is perhaps the most influential in the field due to her view that both women and men had various and complex intentions for using any

---

[1]www.americanspeech.dukejournals.org/content/85/3/315.short

[2]This definition and discussion was found on the website www.mentalfloss.com.

hesitant or more powerful speech. Jennifer Coates (1996) suggested that there was a function at work in the use of these 'feminine' techniques, namely to include the other speaker and to keep the conversation alive – something not associated with insecurity but rather with intelligence. American Deborah Tannen (1995) suggested that women's language was largely based on the role of many women to build rapport through language while men were set up to report. Tannen claimed that women asked men more questions than men asked women, for example, because they had been rehearsed into a specific conversational role and were ultimately more comfortable in conversations by playing this role. Likewise, men were primed to respond to questions rather than to ask them. She believed that both men and women were more comfortable with these roles because of their growing up in distinctly gendered friendship groups. To Tannen, this is why men and women spoke in such gender-specific ways.

In spite of the attention given to gender and language patterns or gendered speech styles throughout the 1990s, language experts today would agree that things said in any conversation depend on many variables, including gender, but also including the participant's age, experience, ethnic background, personality or temperament, job, sexual orientation, as well as the context itself. Janet Holmes' (1995) work on women and men in the workplace strongly linked intention to language use. Holmes claimed that what is intended influences what is said. Her work explored politeness in particular as often aligned with gender – women being more polite, and polite more often, than men. But perhaps politeness is also more aligned with life experiences and the perception of social rewards for politeness rather than gender per se. That is, we may see these tendencies in women but only because we perceive women as having them. The view here is that women are not instinctively or physiologically more polite; rather, they learn to be politer and are rewarded for it. That said, the compelling ingredient of power is always present in some way. How power is enacted in various contexts (by both sexes and across the spectrum of gender identity) is why research into gender and language continues to attract new scholars. How can we understand gendered patterns without reinforcing the view that these are sex-based differences?

More recently, scholars have wondered if discussions on gender differences are helpful at all, because the focus on them supports the possibility that significant differences exist. That is, the exploration presupposes that women and men speak differently, inviting simplistic explanations rather than the more helpful, but also more honestly complex, social constructivism view (defined and expanded on below). But then, why look at gender at all if we believe our roles are so unstable? I think it is because of the infinite possibilities of gender performances that the study of language becomes so meaningful. We are not seeking out differences so to make essentialist claims as much as we are searching for tendencies that are context-driven.

In any event, a key foundation in the field of gender and language use now is the understanding of power relations as a significant aspect to all social interactions. If some people tend to use certain language strategies, such as tag questions or hedges, does this suggest powerlessness? Surely different situations make different demands on different speakers so that there are always many possible reasons for mitigating language devices. Some men (such as academic men, upper-class men, young emo-men) also use what Lakoff identified as 'women's language', suggesting perhaps that these linguistic strategies align with a certain type of person or the possibility of being more class-driven. Some might, regardless of sex, use more stereotypical male bravado language style, such as talking through interruptions, taking more *linguistic space*, or asking fewer questions to other participants. What Robin Lakoff meant in 1975 largely reflected her particular feminist political agenda of interrupting patriarchy by pointing out to women that changing the language could change their world. Her analysis was relevant at the time but is inadequate now in considering the deeper, more complex post-modern variations of speech communities.

It is important to be aware of previous ways language use was defined, analyzed and interpreted in alignment with gender. Focusing on certain sex-preferential language tendencies, such as overlapping speech, questions or silence, may reflect the participants' gendered patterns of interaction, but there remains various possibilities as to the intention or deliberate choices of certain speech behaviors that no theory can fully consider. If a wife asks her silent husband about his day, there are various elements at work to help understand her language use. One can view women as weak or as victims (the deficit/dominance model), or as valued but distinct conversationalists (the difference model). Instead, we can use the sociocultural model – a view of discourses as based on particular choices in particular contexts.

Social Constructionism

There is a persistent and stubborn myth that women use more words per day than men. Mark Peters (2007) indicated that women use about 7000 words a day compared to only 2000 for men. But, '[the discrepancy] is hardly surprising,' says Deborah Cameron, because 'the main influences on how much people speak are contextual – what they're doing and with whom' (quoted in Peters, p. 21). What is the situation? When, why and by whom are words spoken? And where? At home? In the workplace? In the market place? In social contexts? The popular psychology industry loves to pander to such stereotypes in order to sell books.

Social constructionism is concerned with the way our social positions are fluid, negotiable and constantly changing – how they are constantly renegotiated through linguistic and other types of performance. It is the repeated rehearsal of certain ways of speaking that produces gender-differentiated performances. But these stylized gender positions are not fixed. According to social constructionist theory, these positions are challenged and counteracted by the alternative ways in which people are positioned by power relations within a society, according to their age, class, ethnicity, education and sexuality (among other social and psychological variables). People have the potential to enact multiple identities. Social constructionism also recognizes that certain dominant discourses in society (such as gender differentiation) have the power to produce particular identities longer term, which are harder to challenge or resist because of entrenched cultural approval of them (Cameron, 2005).

Scholars like Pia Pichler and Jennifer Coates (2011) use the term *speech style* since very young children participate in very gender-specific subcultures with distinct gender expressions, roles, and expectations, suggesting the socialization process begins very early. The terms 'women's language' and 'men's language' are not particularly helpful, then, in identifying gender patterns because of the reality that gender is relevant across all ages.

From the very early years, young girls face social pressure to be nice while boys are confronted with social pressure to be competitive. How does this general view get transferred from one generation to another? Some of these linguistic choices work to disadvantage girls in certain ways and to disadvantage boys in other ways. Girls seem to be more rehearsed into being relational in their use of language in playing with dolls or in paired groupings, while boys are rehearsed into being more individual through their participation in competitive sports. But both masculine and feminine styles are useful and necessary at various times. Girls and then women may habitually use a conversational style of relationality and come to thrive on it, while boys and men may develop a speech style based on competitiveness. However, using a variety of speech styles would be advantageous to both girls and boys/women and men.

The use of language by any of us depends on where it is being used, why, when, how and by whom. One person's language use will vary widely according to the needs of the social context, in terms of the level of formality required concerning what is being discussed, and in regards to the speakers' relationship and history. For instance, the language one would use in a job interview or when meeting new in-laws is very different from the language used with friends when discussing a film over a drink late on a Saturday night. As such, *sex-preferential speech* can only be helpful to a point because we are more complicated than gendered tendencies.

Sex-preferential tendencies or speech styles are also highly culture-specific. Acquiring them is an important part of learning how to behave as men and women in a particular culture at a particular point in time. And times change. Japanese men's and women's forms of speaking are not as sex-exclusive as they once were. All languages experience sex-preferential tendencies and all speech styles are fluid. What is most likely concerning our gender identities and language patterns is that we are both physiologically formed and socially interactive so that we are many different versions of ourselves, in many different contexts, and with various and altering intentions. Suffice it to say, our use of language reflects our human complexity and our capacity to adjust to circumstances.

Critical Discourse Analysis and Gendered Discourses

What may appear as natural in the everyday lives of women and men is often a result of culturally-produced roles that have become comfortable and, hence, feel 'normal'. We have discussed genderedness as socially constructed; it is worth considering how this happens through language.

To explore the social construction of gender roles in language use, the approach used by linguists is known as *Critical Discourse Analysis* (CDA). We can apply CDA to conversations and in social interactions; 'critical' is used here to mean power relations. CDA is used to examine the way language contributes to social reproduction and social change by exploring power in various linguistic settings. The aim of CDA as a method of framing conversations is to stimulate an awareness of power seen in language use and observe how it emerges as a result of power relations between the participants. As such, CDA is particularly helpful in gender and language studies because of its main concern with, and focus on, power. Sara Mills (2013) sees CDA in

Gender Studies as a way of asking questions about our notions of gender to 'create a productive suspicion of all processes of text interpretation' (p. 21). CDA is a central way researchers in the field of gender and language consider how or when the masculine or feminine is constructed as powerful. If it is the masculine that is viewed and understood as powerful, then this affects the interpretation of conversations in the first place. Conversation participants themselves are likely unaware of the power positions they hold or how their use of language enhances or diminishes this. CDA can frame a conversation so that explorations of genderedness can be considered.

There are many possible discourses in a single conversation (and ways of analyzing them) existing at any one time. Consider a conversation among extended family members at a summer picnic. The language used may include discourses of success ('John has had a promotion at work') or discourses of failure ('Mark has never got over the failure of his first marriage'). In any community, there are various frames/discourses that restrict the conversations and define the power relations and gendered roles.

In the 1970s, the French philosopher and social theorist, Michel Foucault (1972, 1978), considered discourses as structures of both possibility and constraint. Those in the legal profession, for example, use a body of knowledge, practices and social identities in their discourse. Legal discourse defines what is legal and illegal emerging from historically constituted and reinforced by the day-to-day use of certain words, terms and phrases associated with legal matters by lawyers. These specific discourses determine what is possible and what is constrained (not possible) in this field. Foucault believed that knowledge itself could not necessarily reflect any particular truth, but rather it would be the conversation that reflects who has access to this knowledge. Foucault's view is that those who are dominant in any institution, group or community maintain their power and positions of power through discourse; they establish the boundaries and possibilities of belonging through language. For Foucault, it is power that is exercised through the use of certain discourse patterns. Also, counterdiscourses propose alternative versions of social reality, and so these counterdiscourses become important locations for the development of new knowledge and ways of knowing.

Any individual is located within a wide range of positions as a social subject; these are known as *subject positions*. These positions are established in discourse. None of us can exist independently of some kind of discourse; we are constituted in the act of working within various discourses, and we occupy specific social roles through the language we use. We are each a 'constellation of subject positions bestowed by different discourses' (Talbot, 2010: 156). Our subject positions develop in the activities within particular institutions and communities where we participate. For example, by going through a specific training/educational experience one can become a language teacher, as I have done. This position of teacher is an effect of being initiated into an education discourse. We are given, and we take, the words necessary to fully contribute to a certain community in understood ways. Others in my field speak this same language, though subject positions continue to shift throughout our lives. Even within the course of one day, one's subjectivity shifts many times; it is not fixed or even all that coherent. Our subjectivity is diverse and contradictory, displaying remarkable ability to adapt and adjust language use as necessary. Our sense of self is primarily constituted within discourse so that complete self-determination is not possible but, rather, we need others in order to become ourselves – to speak ourselves into communities.

We perform our gendered identities because of the ways we've been rehearsed into specific discourses for particular rewards (or not) of belonging. Consider a young woman who cries when pulled over for speeding. The consequence of her crying may result in a lenient penalty. The same consequence may be unlikely if a young man performed in a similar way. Why? Our interactions with the world are influenced by the ways we are understood by it as well as the ways we have been rewarded by certain behaviors by those around us. If we think of gender as performance, it can keep us from thinking people are passive participants in their own lives or that gender roles are fixed. Whether they are aware of it or not, people have *agency* – the power to choose how to act in any situation. A professional actor is conscious of the role she is playing and behaves accordingly to achieve the best result. As gendered beings, we each do this every day in countless situations.

A critical approach to language (one concerned with power relations) can help us get past the surface of everyday experience and go deeper into understanding of each other. Those who study gender and language look for tensions, contradictions or conflicts found in the working out of power relations in what may go unnoticed or seen as unproblematic. The focus on the relationship of gender and language use is complex, fluid and idiosyncratic. As such, it warrants intense and careful consideration in infinite locations.

All explanations have been valuable and have prompted researchers to ask more questions about the intersection of gender and language use. The social construction of gender is central, though, in understanding the field today. Gender cannot be conceptualized in any simplistic way because there is not a straightforward link between what one says and what one means. Also, the field has largely ignored the study of men until relatively recently, except for its explorations of white, middle-class, heterosexual men in relation to their wives or female business associates. As such, so much more is yet to be explored. My guess is that all new research will support the more complex explanation that gender roles, identities, attitudes and rewards are unstable and ever-changing.

This chapter has explored the relationship of gender and language use, particularly in regards to gender as a performance with various intentions. The next few chapters look at specific aspects of gender in context, namely, in the media, in education, in the workplace, in the church and in personal relationships.

Summing Up

- Language use reflects society's attitudes about men and women, and it creates our attitudes and understandings of gender roles and expectations.
- Various views of gendered language include the theory of deficit and/or dominance, the theory of difference and social constructionism. All views have been located in particular times and all have had some lasting influence on the field.
- Critical Discourse Analysis (CDA) is the usual method used to explore gendered language patterns employed in conversations because it is concerned with power relations; this method generates a necessary and valuable suspicion of the link between what is said and what is meant.

II

Understanding Gender and Language Use in the World

. . . .

II

3

Gender and Language Use in the Media and Technology

. . . .

Gender is the repeated stylization of the body, a set of repeated acts within a rigid regulatory frame which congeal over time to produce the appearance of a 'natural' kind of being.

Judith Butler

The first two chapters (Part I) laid out some necessary understandings in regards to gender studies, feminism, and how gender and language closely connect with each other. The study of gender and language focuses on understanding the relationship between gender and language in various contexts. Modern media are such contexts, and they have much to offer the field of gender and language. It is clear that we live in a world which is increasingly saturated by media and the media's presentations and representations of gender. In particular, one wonders how are the media's 'images and cultural constructions' connected to patterns of inequality, domination and oppression (Gill, 2007: 7)?

Feminist media scholars such as Rosalind Gill (2007) have offered 'rigorous analyses [of media] in the context of ethical and political commitments to creating a more just world' (p. 7). Gill explains how the second-wave feminist campaigns of the 1960s and 1970s faced a significant challenge that earlier women's movements had not experienced: 'a world dominated by media' (p. 9). Second-wave feminists were bombarded with representations of womanhood and gender relations in magazines and on television, in films and on billboards on an unprecedented scale. According to Gill, it is not surprising, under such circumstances, that the media became 'a major focus of feminist research, critique and intervention' (p. 9).

It is not hard to see that gender as social performance aligns with sexuality and sexualization. When it comes to advertising, it is no secret that hyper-masculine and hyper-feminine images sell well. If we agree that society has been patriarchal in its power relations, then we can see how women have been presented and used as an object of men's desires. A prime example of this is the persistent use of attractive women for the purpose of selling cars. In this view, the need for a *heteronormative/heterosexual* gendered identity requires women to see themselves through men's eyes and as consumers of products needed to embellish aspects of themselves that are portrayed as desirable by men. Men are also used as consumers of certain products that enhance the illusion of masculine success (e.g. car advertisements appeal to *semiotics* of the masculine). Conventional kinds of feminine and masculine 'ideals' are strongly shaped by the mass media to produce consumers for specific products. Being feminine and masculine in the heteronormative sense involves particular modes of consumption. As such, advertising creates a need for genderedness: gendered identity is singled out as what needs to be enhanced. When women and men go shopping, they must make decisions on how to genderize themselves based on the products available to them and presented to them as required. Clothing and cosmetic companies in particular depend on heteronormative gendered identities to sell their products. The media are then agents of social control that convey stereotypical and ideological values of women, men, femininity and masculinity.

Gender Identity and the Mass Media

A number of themes connect gender identity and today's media, including the fluidity of our gender identities over time, the decline of the portrayal of traditional gender roles, the idea of gender role models, and the rise of a new 'girl power' (Gauntlett, 2002). Twenty to thirty years ago, analysis of popular media often told researchers that mainstream culture was a backwards-looking force, resistant to social change and able to push people into traditional categories they might be trying to leave behind. Today, researchers are more likely to view mass media as a force for change. The traditional view of a woman as housewife has been replaced by successful and 'raunchy' 'girl power' icons, and the masculine ideals of toughness and self-reliance have been shaken by a new emphasis on men's vulnerability and sensitivities. These alternative ideas and images have created a space for a diversity of identities; yet, they also bring with them new demands and requirements.

Ariel Levy (2005) identified 'raunch culture' and its grip on today's young women in particular as a new site for gender identity formation or performance. She explores the internalizing of misogyny by women themselves who not only participate in heteronormative culture but who also encourage and engage in their own exploitation. Music videos are key sites of this participation. In the 1990s Mary Pipher (1994) identified how adolescent girls internalized society's messages about appearance and thinness. She came down hard on advertisers who push the image of attractive women to impossible standards, profiling isolated body parts (backside, legs, cleavage) to sell perfection and presenting 'woman' as an assembled product. Pipher believed this focus on isolated sections of the body removes any chance to personalize the female form and leads young women to believe that they are only valuable if their body parts look a particular way. For over 20 years these critiques were voiced with little effect. (One such exception is Dove's Real Beauty campaign, for example, where the variety of women's body shapes are celebrated as beautiful).

Presenting a stark contrast to Levy's and Pipher's lament over the sexual demands placed on young women by others and by themselves is David Gauntlett (2002). He sees gender role models in the media as meaningful cultural 'navigation points' for individual members of society. For him, the discourses of 'girl power' concerning sexuality and gender roles are the most prominent expressions of femininity in the mainstream media, and he believes that these expressions can be empowering to many young women.

Regardless of one's view, it is clear that the media disseminate a huge number of messages about identity, including acceptable forms of self-expression, gender, sexuality and lifestyle. At the same time, we each have our own set of diverse feelings on these issues of gender identity, which can change as we move through different life stages. The media's suggestions can be seductive, but only to a point. If the media is sexist, then the culture is as well. Even if we agree that many media sources sustain traditional hierarchical notions of femininity, including newer versions that may appear empowering to young women but simply perpetuate demands on women, we can't ignore the participation and choice that women themselves make: they have agency and they choose to buy the products (Caldas-Coulthard, 1996). We can expect that the specific gender messages will be appropriated by many – maybe even most – but these messages will also be rejected by some. Nevertheless, several researchers and organizations have taken on the role of watchdog when it comes to monitoring the media's gender messages.

For all of us, but especially for children, images and stories help influence the important developmental task of understanding what it means to be human, whether male or female. The *See Jane* organization, a media-watch program, was founded by Academy Award winning actress Geena Davis (*The Accidental Tourist*) in 2004 as a way to explore G-rated films and analyze how male/female characters are marketed. Much of the organization's research has been carried out by Stacy Smith (2006a, 2006b) at the University of Southern California, Los Angeles, and explores G-rated (G for General – family viewing) movies and the portrayal of female and male characters in films marketed to children. Smith and her team explored 101 top-grossing family-rated films released from 1990 through to 2004, analyzing a total of 4,249 speaking characters in the movies, including both animated and live action films. The research found that, overall, three out of four characters (75%) are male, while fewer than one in three (28%) speaking characters are female. Fewer than one in five (17%) characters in crowd scenes are female and more than four out of five (83%) film narrators are male. Smith (2006b) also found that G-rated movies show very few examples of characters as parents or as partners in a marriage or other committed relationship.

In a 2003 American nationwide survey, the Kaiser Family Foundation found that half of all children aged 0–6 watch at least one DVD movie per day. In view of this, G-rated movie DVDs may have an influence on children's early social learning about gender roles because children also tend to watch the same movie over and over. Other studies explore the television viewing habits among children and suggest that gender expectations can become very simplified, skewed and stereotyped (Herrett-Skjellum & Allen, 1996). Since women and girls make up half of the human race, the *See Jane* media watch group in particular believes the presence of a wider variety of female characters in children's earliest experiences with the media is essential for both girls' and boys' development. If both boys and girls see more female characters of all types, we can experience a fuller awareness of the possible ways to be human.

In 2002, the director-actor Rosanna Arquette made a documentary film called *Searching for Debra Winger* about how hard it is to be a female actor in Hollywood. She wanted to answer the question: can a woman have both her art and a life? She interviewed a wide range of very successful Hollywood women, including Jane Fonda, Meg Ryan, Sharon Stone and Vanessa Redgrave. Eventually, Arquette's search led her to the home of Debra Winger herself, an Academy Award nominee who stopped making films mid-career.

Winger offered some insight into her disappearance from the silver screen, saying that she simply never really liked acting anyway. However, the other actors interviewed along the way say much more about how difficult, even impossible, it is to have both an acting career and a personal life as a woman: the demands on both personal time and appearance are unrelenting. All participants in the documentary mention the lack of roles available for women over 40 in particular and the use of younger women in roles within a very narrow definition of attractiveness: young, skinny, long hair, clear skin, perfect teeth. The demands are exhausting – if not impossible – for female actors. If women in Hollywood resist the ideal, the industry can find many others who will fit the ideal. As such, expertise and talent that grow with age are not rewarded as much as youth and youthful beauty. That said, the last 15 years have seen the emergence of women over 40 succeeding in film and television as well as featured in beauty advertisements. Perhaps this shift is related to the aging of *baby-boomers* themselves and, thus, the industry is keeping up with the need to appeal to a greater number of people who are growing older.

Advertising Gender

In modern industrial societies, gender identities are heavily determined by capitalist social conditions. This is an important point to understand. At the advent of television in the 1950s, women, in their roles as wives and mothers, were often responsible for most of the shopping. As a result, women became caught up in what is called *consumer femininity* – something that women participate in to feminize themselves and/or to perform traditional female roles. The assumption seemed to be that women in western society were to buy certain products; to do so, they had to buy into the need for the product. Advertisements from this time depicted housewives in the kitchen, for example, marveling at a new kitchen appliance. Consumer culture also affects men and their *consumer masculinity* when it came to advertising cars or male cologne. *Consumer gender* enters our daily relationships with the world and is a major influence on our patterns of behavior in society, including at work, in the home, and in our friendships and relationships with others. Consumer gender is a construction used by the mass media in which we co-participate. We spend our time and money to construct ourselves into certain acceptable versions of men or women. These gender identities require much effort and expense on the part of individuals, while generating incredible profits for industries.

Rosalind Gill (2007) explores the construction of gender identities in media discourse, noting that it is a complicated process. Her insights include the compelling view that femininities and masculinities are established, reinforced and increasingly played with more and more use of irony. In fact, many media scholars now see irony as increasingly displayed in media and are using irony as a key term in the vocabulary of media critique. Irony here is the use of 'knowingly ridiculous representations that are based on the assumption that it's "silly to be sexist"' (Gill, 2007: 111). Is it possible that feminist critiques have influenced media so extensively that they have transformed its representations of identity, subjectivity and desires resulting in the media using irony as a way of both accepting the critique and for the continued purpose of selling products as gender-specific? Gender in the media exists in relation to an assumed audience so that, while media producers construct or inverse an *ideal*, consumers position themselves in relation to that ideal (Fairclough, 1992). This ideal is particularly visible in women's and men's magazines where the creation and establishment of femininity or masculinity defines what is 'normal' – even as this 'normal' becomes increasingly ironic. Mass media are propelled by the market and its views and values. The market wants to understand consumers, not because it cares for them, but because the sale is their central virtue. The relationship of sellers and buyers is central to capitalism as well as to neoliberalism: making money is the chief goal, and it is the responsibility of an individual person to make themselves 'successful'. As such, advertising expands on ideals and/or values and creates a deeper need for a certain product as necessary for success.

It is critical to understand that the media images of female beauty are unattainable for most women. The influential work of Jean Kilbourne (2000) has been helpful. She reports that women's magazines have 10 and a half times more advertisements and articles promoting weight loss than do men's magazines, and over 75 of women's magazines' covers include at least one message about how to change a woman's bodily appearance. Twenty years ago, the average model weighed 8% less than the average woman, but today's models weigh 23% less. The barrage of messages about thinness, dieting and beauty tells ordinary women that they are always in need of adjustment. Women internalize these stereotypes and judge themselves and others harshly because of this (Kilbourne, 2000).

Jean Kilbourne's work points out the dreamlike promise of advertising that leaves women in particular never satisfied: we can always improve something. The barrage of advertising (some 3,000 advertisements produced per day) affects young people especially, creating an 'addictive mentality' concerning 'self-improvement' that often continues throughout life. Why are standards of beauty being imposed on women, the majority of whom are naturally larger and older than any of the models? It is because, by presenting an ideal difficult to achieve and maintain, the cosmetic and diet industries are assured of growth and profits. Women who are required to be insecure about their bodies are more likely to buy beauty products, new clothes and diet aids, even if exposure to images of thin, young, air-brushed female bodies is linked to depression and loss of self-esteem. Women are required to do whatever is necessary to conform to 'acceptable' images of femininity.

The demands on men may be as great as those placed on women, but their hypothetical rewards are more empowering. They 'get to be' rich and powerful, while all that women can hope for is to be physically appealing and, hopefully, very thin. Although much contemporary research on masculinity in the media has focused on violence in TV and film, some research has examined the portrayal of masculinity in men's magazines such as *Maxim*, *GQ* and *Esquire*. These magazines also play a part in defining what it means to be a modern man through the same use of a *synthetic gender community*.

Media Discourse

Though there are magazines and television programming targeted specifically at men, the range of media targeted at women is staggering and long-standing: fashion magazines, women's homemaking magazines, celebrity magazines, women's television networks, daytime talk shows, daytime soap-operas, food channels. The question here is why does being a woman require so many products? Lia Litosseliti (2006) lists several women's magazines in the UK, each connecting with an 'ideal' magazine audience where women are young, white, able-bodied, middle-class, heterosexual and conventionally attractive. In each case, the magazine uses phrases to brand itself in a way that shows its connection to its female audience. Consider the use of language as found on the covers of these magazines in the UK, particularly in regards to identity, subjectivity and desire. Do you see any differences in the way the magazines brand themselves?

Cosmopolitan	The World's No. 1 magazine for young women
She	For women who know what they want
B	Everything you want
Woman's Own	For the way you live your life and the way you'd like to
Company	For your freedom years
Minx	For girls with a lust for life
Femina (India)	For the woman of substance
Executive woman	For women who really do mean business
Wench	Where women are, where they are going, and where they should be already

(Litosseliti, 2006: 97)

Clearly, the branding highlights the presence of neoliberalism, as the messages underscore the demand and desire for success. The messages present the view that it's in the hands of individual women to improve themselves, to make their lives 'successful'. Litosseliti highlights the use of personal pronouns ('you', 'your', 'we') as a common feature used in media that assumes and thereby creates a relationship between manufacturer and consumer (i.e. 'Everything *you* want' and that the magazine can tell you). The use of personal phrases in editorials (such as 'most of us' or 'we've all done it') makes connections with a reader that creates a sense of solidarity. Mary Talbot (1995) called this *synthetic sisterhood*. This is an artificial construction of a gender-centered community located in an ideal setting where economic or social differences are not made explicit. As a result, the message is that any woman can imagine herself as part of the successful sisterhood. Any woman can live an 'ideal' successful life. What matters is that consumers feel a kindred connection and, hence, there is an establishment of a loyal consumer relationship: women who read these magazines subscribe to its values and assumptions of gender performances. Men's products and advertising work in a similar way: a community is assumed, then established, and then a relationship emerges where certain key products are highlighted as enhancing the gender identity of its consumers as ways of belonging to the desired group.

Talbot (1995) was critical of this consumer femininity/masculinity because of the way in which it manipulates women into assuming the role of helpless, gullible consumers and men into presenting themselves as sex-crazed and car-loving. To belong, women must look a certain way (and for each new season) and share common values and tastes; likewise, men must perform masculinity in a particular way. Women are rehearsed into a certain kind of femininity for the sake of a consumer-driven market, as are men and their masculinity. Women seek out participation in gender communities and then are trapped by them. One key example of this is the *O* magazine. Each issue is a site for connection with their 'buddy' Oprah who shares her favorite things – books, advice and fashion features each month. To belong to this 'Oprah community' requires a shared aesthetic and value system regarding self-improvement and 'living your best life'.

Most of the mainline, popular magazines, television shows and movies assume a heterosexual audience and, therefore, reinforce the presupposition that women and men are biologically different. As a direct result, the assumption reinforces the position that both sexes are not complex or ambiguous but are easy to understand and are generalizable. The media polarizes men and women, boys and girls in terms of values, behaviors and styles: men are like this while women are like that. This in turn influences our views of the sexes; though they have been presented to us as stereotypes, we begin to accept those generalizations as the 'norm' against which we judge ourselves and others. For example, we see the Old Spice man as a 'norm', rather than an image of men manipulated for the sake of the sale. Even with newer men's lifestyle magazines that began to emerge in the 1990s and with the rise of masculinities studies, there are still deep assumptions about gender performances concerning masculinities. It's worth considering that the 'new man' has been created as a version of masculinity that is concerned with relationships, fashion, health, fitness and appearance. This 'new man' is in some ways a positive development, but it is also a confusing one. On the one hand, he is aligned with traditional masculinity based on male success, wealth, power and heterosexual desire while, at the same time, he is also connected to progressive approaches to relationships and family life. The presentation of contradiction and complexity is positive, but a tension exists between the celebration of various representations of heterosexual masculinity and the promotion of new standards of beauty and grooming. In either representation, gender identity is still used to create desire, need and a version of 'success' that requires participation in consumer culture.

Several recent examples highlight the contradictory nature of gender in the media. Comedy shows like Sarah Haskins' *Target Women* (2013) program on the Comedy Network successfully expose the contradictions. Her short, ten-minute vignettes focus on advertising; each episode looks at current ads, and she uses irony to expose the contradictions. In one particular episode, she focuses on how yogurt is portrayed as a woman's food and one that brings a woman complete health and deep satisfaction that replaces sexual longing for a man with a craving for yogurt.

Most advertisements are targeted to a specific consumer and are connected to programming that is demographically based. Advertisements during the airing of a large sporting event differ significantly from those appearing during a morning television program directed at women. The images in magazines or in advertisements create a fantasy world where power is achieved through clothes, a favorite beverage, cosmetics or social setting – in short, it is through the use of the product that gender is identified and developed. It is fair to say that gender manipulation is central to advertising and the media discourse which surrounds it. One recent example of such manipulation is found in *The Guardian's* (2016) report on Boots Drug Store in the UK selling pink razors to women for more money than the same razors in blue that were being sold to men.

Advertisements have also contributed to the perceived 'crisis of masculinity' discourse, where men are portrayed not only as victims of feminism but also as a sex caught in a whirlwind of possibilities about what it is to be a man. The 'crisis of masculinity' discourse suggests that media have appropriated the earlier feminist discourse of deficit/dominance to promote the male experience as being deficient and/or dominated by women. Lazar (2005) refers to this as a discourse of 'popular post-feminism' or a 'global neo-liberal discourse of post-feminism', which states that now that certain gains for women have been made, feminism has achieved its purpose and should therefore be dropped, out of a concern for the apparent crisis of masculinity. These constructions of alleged equality, or even a reversal of gender roles and power, obscure actual and remaining gender inequalities and the consistent inequalities that will always plague both women's and men's life experiences. Until our societies can move beyond 'zero-sum games' where there can only be one winner, we are stuck with the deficit-dominance-different debates.

Talk Shows, the News, TV and Film

It is doubtful that news media producers are concerned about or interested in the implications of gender representations beyond an investment in newsworthy gender-related stories (e.g. Bruce/Caitlyn Jenner, high-profile celebrities' domestic abuse cases, etc.). Sara Mills (2003) critiques how media texts are authored and how different criteria influences what is reported and how. Both talk shows and news broadcasts are fascinating sites for gender studies.

Many scholars have described a variety of factors for the selection of primary news items. Media and Cultural Studies analyses since the 1980s have turned attention to how audiences use texts; that said, the use of CDA (Critical Discourse Analysis) in a search for genderedness can be tricky. Media has a range of meanings, a range of audiences, and a range of interpretations. Successful programming connects with specific target audiences – those which align with particular attitudes and life experiences. These target audiences are often gender-based. Take, for example, the popular *Oprah Winfrey Show*, that was watched by over 6 million viewers a day for 25 years from 1986 to 2011. This talk show connected with middle-class women who were concerned about their families, their relationships with spouses and friends, their appearance, and home decorating – all stereotypical concerns of women. Do such shows reveal attitudes already out there or promote concerns and create a market niche? It is likely both. *The Oprah Winfrey Show* was one of the most successful daytime programs for women, and it was based on an assumed need that women want to improve themselves.

The media serves as both a mirror and a tool of gender stereotyping, so it is worth reflecting on its power to coerce and manipulate. In film studies, the development of the Bechdel test, named after the American cartoonist Alison Bechdel (whose comic strip *Dykes to watch out for* first appeared in 1985), has become a quick way to search out sexism in movies (Bechdel, 1986). The test has become more widely discussed in the 21st century than it ever was in the mid-1980s. The test explores a work of fiction to see if it features at least two women who talk to each other about something other than a man. It is used as an indicator of the presence (or absence) of women in film or television and calls attention to gender inequality and sexism as foundational to many popular storylines. According to a 2014 study by the Geena Davis Institute (the See Jane organization) on Gender in the Media, in 120 films made worldwide from 2010 to 2013, only 31% of named characters were women; only 23% of the films had a female protagonist or co-protagonist and only 7% of directors were women. Looking at 700 top-grossing films from 2007 to 2014, Davis's research group found that only 30% of the speaking characters were female. In addition, female characters have been portrayed as involved in sex twice as often as men, while scenes with explicit sexual content have increased (not decreased) over time. Violence against women in film has increased dramatically in the past 10 years in particular. Since 2010 the Bechdel test has been understood as the standard by which feminist critics judge television, movies, books and other media (Ulaby, 2008).

By 2013, it had become 'a household phrase, common shorthand to capture whether a film is woman-friendly.' The value of the test is not about the discrepancies in representation of the sexes but it helps articulate something about the missing depth in women's characters and the range of concerns regarding women. The website www.bechdeltest.com is a user-edited database of some 5,000 films classified by whether or not they pass the test. As of 2015, some 55% of these films passed. Interesting to note: *Sex and the City* (a television show which ran on HBO from 1998 until 2004) failed the Bechdel test, since the women in the show talked mainly about men.

In April 2016, Polygraph-Film Dialogue (found at http://polygraph.cool/films/) reported that the majority of dialogue in 22 out of 30 Disney films to date is male. Even in films with female leads, like *Mulan*, the dialogue 'swings male'. Mushu, Mulan's protector dragon, for example, has 50% more words of dialogue than Mulan herself. A plot can center around a character even if the dialogue doesn't reflect this. The researchers at Polygraph searched screenplays and mapped characters with at least 100 words of dialogue, though there are weaknesses with the methodology since films can change quite a bit from 'script to screen'. As such, each screenplay they reviewed had at least 90% of its lines characterized by gender. Across thousands of films in their dataset, it was hard for them to 'find a subset that didn't over-index male'.

> Even romantic comedies have dialogue that is, on average, 58% male. For example, *Pretty Woman* and *10 Things I Hate About You* both have lead women (i.e., characters with the most amount of dialogue). But the overall dialogue for both films is 52% male, due to the number of male supporting characters (online).

In only 22% of the films Polygraph researchers explored did actresses have the most amount of dialogue (i.e. they were the lead character). Women are more likely to speak less than men. They lament that women occupy at least two of the top three roles in a film in only 18% of Hollywood films, while 'that same scenario for men occurs in about 82% of films'. Some critics of the Bechdel test say that some films fail due to 'historical reasons', but an exploration of actual dialogue (in particular, words spoken) gives a good indication of sexism in major motion pictures. Sexism is also seen in the age of women and men actors, with fewer words spoken by women over 40 and increasingly more words spoken by men over 40. Their website continues to monitor Hollywood films in this way.

Technology as Mediated Community

All around the world, the internet and mobile phones have transformed how humans connect. Technology has also, however, led to a widening and perhaps even surprising gender gap. For much of the world, men control the *information revolution* that helps to educate, inform and empower those with access to technology. Some of the key topics in regards to gender in the information revolution include the gendered use of technology, computer gaming and the limits of technology in creating an equitable society.

We are all communicators. The emergence of various technologies has opened up our capacity to connect more frequently with each other. The usual barriers of distance, expense and ability are gone. With a click of a button, we are instantly connected with another human being and can access an infinite variety of websites, blogs, forums and news media. Electronically *mediated* communication has transformed our notion of the relationship between place and community. In contrast with face-to-face communication or even static media (i.e. print), a greater proportion of our communicative acts are now taking place via electronic media. Electronic media include any medium of communication that requires electricity and/ or digital encoding such as television, radio, internet, fax, DVD, email, instant messaging, websites, Twitter, Instagram, text messages and audio/video including Facebook and Skype. The list seems endless. These new forms of community connectivity have led to new conceptualizations of community as well as new forums in which to explore gender and language.

Technology has advanced so very quickly that researchers have a hard time keeping up with the roles new technologies may play in the human experience. How have technologies changed us? How has human society adjusted to the new ways of connecting? How are gender and language inter-secting in these new ways of communicating? Such research areas (including gendered performance on Facebook or the effect of Facebook on young women and men) invite newer and newer conceptualizations of gender in society. The new mediated communities rely on language to connect them; in fact, the whole enterprise is based on the use of words and symbols. Fashion blogs, feminist blogs, dating sites and YouTube, to name just a few, are examples of new mediated communities; there is now a whole variety of communities that did not exist before communicative technology innovations emerged in the 1990s.

One can consider whether gender 'differences' in attitudes concerning privacy issues exist. Personal sharing and other behaviors on social networks seem to suggest this is so, especially as newer and newer sites of connection also come with more and more gender performances, while privacy laws and government regulation have been slow to respond.

Researchers (e.g. Totten & Berbary, 2015) explore deeply the intersections of identities on the world wide web. For example, how do Black men negotiate their identities online? What about young girls in South America? How did gender play a role in the Arab Spring? There are a whole host of possible areas of inquiry. As the world adjusts to technological changes in communication, so do the communities.

Misogynistic Abuse

Social networking websites (Twitter, Facebook, etc.) have also provided a new platform for gender discrimination, sexism and misogyny. Unprecedented public vitriol against women, as seen on Twitter, for example, exposes highly gender-specific, violent threats to 'silence' women with a public voice, especially when they use it to discuss 'gender issues'. Women such as Caroline Criado-Perez (2013) have exposed the sustained harassment on Twitter, including threats made to women of rape or murder. In her own case, she was receiving 50 such threats an hour over several weeks after her campaign to put a woman on a British bank note was successful. (The image of Jane Austen now appears on the £10 note.)

Criado-Perez is certainly not the only one to find such misogynistic abuse on Twitter and Facebook. Such abuse seems to be a well-known reality for women with a presence on the web, particularly if they have an opinion that they are willing to put out there. In Criado-Perez's view, 'men get attacked because they've said or done something someone doesn't like, whereas women get attacked because they are visible' (quoted in Driscoll, 2013).

Gaming and a Non-Gendered Community

More and more academic studies are exploring how individual differences in the consumption of computer games intersect with gender.

American scholar Pam Royse and her colleagues (2007) focus their research on women and computer games. They put forward three levels of game consumption for women. One is the intense high-level gamers who are focused on mastery of the game, something based on skill and competition. Second level moderate users play for pleasure, and use gaming for entertainment and amusement. The third level is the non-gamers who express strong criticisms about game-playing and gaming culture. There is a whole range of how girls and women interact with computer gaming, and it may surprise some readers to hear that many girls and women do connect with gaming at high levels. Gaming is not just for boys and men.

Michele Zorrilla (2013), an emerging feminist researcher, identified video games as a global form of sport, entertainment and education. She particularly highlights the growing platforms and growing appreciation for gaming that is at the center of the industry's marketing. She interviewed professionals in both public relations firms and gaming studios to identify key challenges to today's industry (such as time, knowledge, adaptability, etc.). She highlights how there are products to sell and how gender and sexuality are key ingredients to the sale of various technologies.

Since video games first entered the market in the 1970s, there has been an influx of thousands of games the world over. Gaming's reach is immense. Williams and colleagues (2009) research the violence and attitudes towards women and minorities in particular. He says it's critical to appreciate the variety of content and context, and he believes that seeing computer gaming as one entity is 'the equivalent of assuming that all television, radio or motion picture use is the same' (p. 70). Instead, the variety is central in understanding the entirety.

Researchers apply *cultivation theory* to the effect television and films have on society and how 'media consumption cultivates in us a distorted perception of the world we live in, making [life] seem more like television portrays it, than it is in real life' (Ivy & Backlund, 2008: 99). Video games are a key part of this 'cultivation'. Of concern to feminist scholars is the gender representations within many video games of how men and women are depicted differently concerning competence, physical attributes, role in the game and physical representation (in terms of body, attire, etc.). Current findings concerning gender representation in video games support past findings regarding males as more represented in media in general. As in film, there are more males represented than females by approximately 3:1 (577 male characters to 196 female characters) (Williams *et al.*, 2009: 824). Other research (like Jansz & Martis, 2007) suggests the trend may be changing, but no significant shifts have yet been detected. Some games provide users with the ability to choose character gender representation (such as The Sims 2) but even then, there are more male characters selected in these games (60% to 40%).

Going further, Burgess *et al.* (2007) suggest:

> females would be more likely to share their primary status with a primary male. Even with a primary female character, the presence of a primary male implied that the female was only allowed to be an important part of the game because the male was there with her. The male could serve as protector, guide, or actually perform most of the action while the female served as a sidekick. (p. 425)

Whether this is accurate or not, video games are often criticized for their negative and/or violent effects on users, and most studies over the years support this: video games do cultivate violence and aggression in those who play them. That said, researchers like Shibuya *et al.* (2008) find that there is an increase in male aggression with video gaming but not so in females. Anderson and Bushman's (2001) work is significant here. The results of their meta-analysis of all relevant studies points to violent video games 'regardless of whether the game rewards or punishes violence, increases aggressive affect' (p. 887) as a factor in increased levels of violence in both males and females.

A host of researchers also claim that viewing violent images of male aggression behavior and/or sexually exploitative images of females is disastrous for everyone. Others (e.g. Williams & Skoric, 2005) find no link whatsoever between video game play and aggressive sexual thoughts and behaviors. Instead, they cite age as the key variable. It is older participants who can be more strongly influenced by game play; they also argue with friends more than younger counterparts. Why? It seems those who are younger (such as those who are 10-12 years old) have grown up with such technologies and, therefore, are less intensely involved: an immunity is built in. Those over 40, whose exposure to video games came later in their lives, may be the most affected by video game violence and the misogyny the game can promote.

Interesting findings are emerging regarding sex/gender patterns in relation to computer games. Matthew Eastin's (2006) analysis on female violence based on *avatar gender* found that women playing female characters experienced *greater* aggression in the game than when they were playing male characters. Jackson *et al.* (2009) found that boys, regardless of race or other sociocultural variables, played more video games than girls, and this was associated with a lower self-concept and self-esteem in young men. They wondered if this was due to the highly sexualized nature and masculine body image ideals that they are unable to match in real life, whereas girls don't experience lower self-concept and self-esteem when playing those same games. Regardless of debates that question the socialization of video games, it may well be that content, context and personal circumstances each play a part and, hence, the effects are too varied to be generalizable in any real way concerning gender communities and gender roles and behaviors.

Girls and Technology

Claire Charles (2007) used Judith Butler's (1990) notion of performativity to investigate the role of digital technologies in what she calls 'girling' (processes of gendered subjectification) in a private all-girls school. This gender-specific location reveals the potential of student-led constructions and explorations of 'femininity' in the form of self-promotional texts in which young femininity is regulated by discourses of 'girl power'.

In many ways the first era of the internet has opened up new possibilities of self-identity work (including empowering women) while simultaneously reinforcing stereotypes that have perpetuated sexist, racist and even terrorist views. The American non-profit organization, Girls Who Code, and many other educational organizations and institutions highlight the disconnect between girls' achievement and performance in schools and the discouraging figure that only 0.4% of high school girls select computer science as a college major, even while 74% of American girls express interest in STEM (Science, Technology, Engineering and Mathematics). These numbers closely match other Western nations. While more and more young women go to college and university (now 57% of the total number of students), only 12% of computer science degrees are awarded to women (see www.girlswhocode.org).

There's another, and perhaps more disturbing, statistic: while 12–18% of current computer science graduates are women, in 1984 they represented 37%. Why such a drop rather than an increase of women in computer science? One wonders if there have been any lasting gains achieved by the women's movement over the past 30 years or if, instead, there have been significant setbacks. Have progressive attitudes been halted (or even reversed) because of the gender discrepancies now experienced in computer use, computer skills, or working and owning tech businesses? If so, why would this be? Could it be partly the way computers were initially sold as gendered toys to boys (rather than to girls) in the 1980s? And how has language contributed to the male-dominated world of technology? Linguists are searching out some possibilities when it comes to more and more (not less and less) sexist messages in relation to technology. The increasing disparity is a worrying trend as the world grows in its reliance on computers and technologies that, ultimately, seem designed *by* men and, for the most part, *for* them.

Summing Up

- Conventional kinds of feminine and masculine appearance are shaped by the mass media to produce consumers for various products. As such, consumer gender is intricately connected to our gendered identities.
- Consumer femininity and consumer masculinity is something we participate in to genderize ourselves; this participation influences our daily relationships and is a major part of our pattern of behavior at work, at home and in our friendship groups.
- Though men can be objectified in media images, the manipulation of women is far more destructive because media images present women as often helpless, gullible and even invisible, thus promoting a cultural misogyny that is deeply embedded.

4

Gender and Language Use in Education

. . . .

We cannot all succeed when half of us are held back.

Malala Yousafzai

The vast area of education is of concern to many of us around the world. Recent statistics reveal how sex discrimination in the education system affects both boys/men and girls/women during and after their education experiences. More men are likely to be literate on a global average (100 men to 88 women), although there are more women in higher education in the Organisation for Economic Co-operation and Development (OECD) countries. In the US in particular, girls are significantly ahead of boys in writing ability at all levels (K-12), with boys slightly ahead of girls in mathematical ability.

Because education is an institution of social and cultural reproduction, the existing patterns of gender inequality are reproduced within schools through both formal and informal processes. In particular, classrooms and the surrounding school culture are important settings for the foundations of social behavior. The construction of one's gender identity and the resulting relationship with the world is rehearsed day in and day out inside schools. Thus, gender, language use and education are inevitably and intimately connected. This chapter explores the relationship of gender and achievement, gender and teacher behavior, as well as gender performances inside classrooms.

Gender, Achievement, the Hidden Curriculum and Linguistic Space

There is a substantial and wide-ranging body of research connecting gender with achievement. Much work was done in the 1980s and 1990s concerning gender 'differences' in the classroom, particularly as regarding class participation, speaking up in class and educational attainment levels. Certainly, recent research has marked a shift away from gender generalizations or gender differences to examine the discourses and the various gender and sexual identities that are at work in various educational settings. A search for differences seems limited while an exploration of various contexts seems to offer more nuanced understandings.

The specific structures surrounding classrooms and classroom life are of particular interest to the study of gender and language use. Many researchers have offered various pieces to the puzzle. For example, the work of Rebecca Oxford (1994) on gender differences in language classrooms focused on the particular learning styles noted in females and on the particular learning strategies often employed by girls in school. After discussion of the many possible gender differences (such as subjectivity or objectivity, field dependence or independence, reflection or sensory preference) she put forward a conclusion:

> Anatomy is not destiny, as Freud suggested, but a learner's sex—or, more likely, gender—can have profound effects on the ways that learners approach language learning, ways which may in turn affect proficiency. (p. 146)

The hidden curriculum also promotes discrimination in the educational system. It refers to the idea that teachers interact with and teach their students in a way that reinforces relations of gender (as well as race and social class). For example, teachers may give more attention to boys, thus encouraging them to speak up in class and become more social. Conversely, girls may become quieter and learn that they should be passive and defer to their male classmates. Samuel Bowles and Herbert Gintis (2011) suggest the correspondence principle, where girls may be encouraged to learn skills valued in female-dominated fields, while boys might learn leadership skills for male-dominated occupations. Sex discrimination in the classroom both at high school and college have also resulted in women not being prepared or qualified to pursue more prestigious, high-paying occupations. Sex discrimination in education has resulted in grown women being more passive, quiet and less assertive because of the effects of the hidden curriculum.

One of the themes that ran through the early work of Valerie Walkerdine (1990) is that all classrooms are sites of some gender struggle. At the time, she saw classrooms as sites of frequent passive and silent struggles on the part of many girls. With the emergence of masculinities study in education, this idea could be expanded on to say that classrooms are sites of gender identity formation for all children. Struggles to participate may exist because of the power relations experienced more generally. The classrooms in Walkerdine's research revealed offensive and at times aggressive discourse on the part of male students to their female teachers and female classmates. Other studies have also found maleness to be a major indicator of power and legitimacy as demonstrated through certain gendered speech practices, both inside classrooms and on school playgrounds. Research that has focused on primary classrooms (such as nursery schools, reception classes, kindergartens) has explored discourse used in the very early years. Brownhill *et al.* (2015) are currently researching masculinities in early education. Their study is premised on the view that gender is formed early in the human experience. Earlier studies like Geoffrey Short and Bruce Carrington's (1990) research of young children's attitudes also suggested the possibility that gender roles and expectations are prescribed early in life, are accepted by children, and appear relatively stable; that is, the children viewed gender as a fixed element of themselves and others by the age of five. When the children in their study were asked explicitly about gender roles, they responded with traditional gender stereotyping comments (such as, 'mommies cook', 'daddies build things'); a significant number of children spoke of the traditional gender roles as 'natural' and permanent characteristics.

Some roles or habits in classrooms seem to reflect the patriarchy outside the classroom, in a society that sees more power being equated to the male or the masculine and less power associated with the female or the feminine. A lack of self-esteem among many girls may be the main point of concern when considering gender in the classroom, particularly in secondary schooling. But, again, more recent research explores masculinities and the heteronormativity of schools, enlarging the scope. Girls and boys tend to describe themselves as fundamentally different from each of their classmates' description of themselves. Research in this area suggests that both boys and girls participate in creating the existing power differences and that they likely do this as a way of belonging to their various classroom communities.

Observational studies have examined what children do in classrooms when selecting certain toys or books – girls select more stereotypical feminine items, such as dolls, and boys select more stereotypical masculine items, such as trucks and blocks. Such studies have also looked at which stories teachers read to children and how gender is presented in these stories – who is the main character? Who are the antagonists? These items often align with gender stereotypes. Also, what in the school culture itself is seen in special events and the language used? The earlier interactional analysis work of

Nicholas Flanders (1970) found that the teacher-dominated approaches established in most classrooms limit student contributions in general and perhaps female contributions in particular, because student contributions rely on report-style discussions – something traditionally more comfortable for boys to perform.

Michael Gurian and Kathy Stevens (2005) published *The Minds of Boys: Saving Our Sons from Falling Behind in School and Life*. Their ideas follow a host of books on the similar theme of 'saving' the boys. But Dan Kindlon and Michael Thompson's (1999) *Raising Cain: Protecting the Emotional Life of Boys* and William Pollack's (1998) *Real Boys: Rescuing our Sons from the Myths of Boyhood* are quite different. These discussions more successfully problematize gendered expectations of boys while the other publications listed above join a number of books that appeal to worries that boys are the new failures and, thus, it is imperative to equip boys in schools to be strong and able to succeed. The 'crisis' discourse of lower grades, drop-out rates, and lower and later reading levels among boys reinforces the necessity to keep boys 'on top' by appealing to their 'male learning style' and their more physical, aggressive and competitive traits – an essentialist view of masculinity. Such ideas raise the contradictions between feminist educational discourses. The feminist educational discourses connect with the vulnerability concerning children. Our emotional ties to our children are powerful sites of desire: we have dreams, often gendered dreams, for our sons and daughters.

Kindlon and Thompson's (1999) *Raising Cain* taps into the gendered ways we treat boys and how this treatment seems to align with the higher risk for suicide, alcohol and drug abuse, violence and loneliness. They explore various explanations for these tendencies, including 'mother blame' and 'boy biology'; they settle on the way society trains boys to be emotionally disengaged. We see this in the promotion of video games, violent movies and thrill-seeking sports that remove boys from more connected relationships. Kindlon and Thompson call this the 'culture of cruelty', in which boys receive little (if any) encouragement to develop qualities such as compassion, sensitivity and warmth. Boys have limited emotional literacy because we, as a society, demand a particular type of masculinity that is success driven and relationally vacant. William Pollack (1998) calls this 'the Boy Code' – our demand that boys suppress or cover up their emotions.

The messages (or discourses) are contradictory within educational discussions. On one hand, feminist literature says girls are ignored, yet they have a much higher success rate educationally. On the other hand, boys are given far more attention and resources, yet they continue to be failures. Why? Judith

Baxter (2003) responds to this. Drawing on her perceptions of post-feminism, she sees these realities as evidence of the individuality at work in each context. We make choices, consciously or otherwise, to position ourselves in fluid identities and behave in ways we are expected to by the context we're in.

What Do We Call the Toilets?

A unisex public toilet or a gender-neutral public toilet/restroom/washroom or all-gender restrooms are public toilets that people of any gender or gender identity may use. Dalhousie University in Canada (2014) defines a gender-neutral washroom as 'one where the signage is visibly identified with open, inclusive language, not just male or female [...]. Some people are not comfortable using male or female-designated.' As schools adjust to more visibility of LGBTQ students in educational institutions, school governing bodies need policies in place to accommodate students' needs and assure their well-being. New schools can be built with single-user all-gender restrooms. In addition to offering privacy for users, these can be cost- and space-efficient. These unisex restrooms are already used on airplanes or trains. Changing already existing schools' structure to create safe unisex toilets may be challenging. Transgender advocacy groups promote all-gender washrooms/restrooms/toilets, believing they eliminate gender-based bullying that happens in big public washrooms where stalls are lined up. All-gender washrooms are helpful for students whose gender identities may be in flux; sharing washroom space may be quite difficult for them. Changing of signage for unisex toilets is happening in many universities and public buildings in the UK and Canada. The city of Vancouver was among the first cities to change building codes to require gender-neutral facilities, basing this decision on human rights. In Vancouver, Canada, doors are often simply labeled 'washroom' (Judd, 2014). Religious schools, however, have difficulty in offering gender-neutral facilities because of traditionally clear divides between females and males.

The Teacher as Gender Coach; Classrooms as Gender Stage

Many studies have confirmed that teachers seem unaware that they treat boys and girls differently and even disbelieve the evidence when confronted with it. Indeed, it may be common for teachers to defend their actual practices with a sincere disclaimer that they treat them all the same. Because classrooms are filled with language, students are engaged with language for most of the day. If there are marked and consistent patterns in the ways boys and girls participate in their classrooms, what are these tendencies and what are the implications? In their early work, Dale Spender and Elizabeth Sarah (1980/1990) believed that girls were the ones who were

> 'learning how to lose' at the game of education, undemanding of teacher time, passive, background observers to boys' active learning, ... and to strive for success within traditional, domestic, nurturing careers. (p. 27)

The zero-sum game of gender and achievement (that is, that one gender must win and one must lose) is on the wane. Gender classifications also index sex, but there are other social variables, such as race. Much of the 1960s Civil Rights Movement was concerned with desegregation of schools. We now understand that regardless of test scores or academic achievement, determining the 'success' of any girl or boy, of any sexual identity, ethnic background and social class remains complex and contradictory. Higher test scores on the part of girls do not seem to correlate with high academic achievement or to be an indication of high success later in life (Davies, 1999). Even when girls appear to 'win' at the education game, they lose out on long-term achievement or leadership roles later in life.

It has also been argued that teacher attitudes toward gender within education have historical, structural and ideological roots, and that systemic attitudes toward gender are revealed in 'teacher talk' (Thornborrow, 2014). Such studies indicate gender discrimination in classrooms exists largely at a covert level (Delamont, 2012; McKnight, 2015). Gender discrimination in classrooms is hard to identify because teachers seem to 'know what teaching is' not from teacher training programs (no matter how enlightened) but from their own previous classroom experiences as students; they thus largely perpetuate accepted attitudes from their past. As a result, the majority of primary teachers do not regard gender as relevant. Rather, primary and kindergarten teachers feel that they treat all children the same – as unique 'individuals' rather than as gendered characters. With blinkers on their eyes, gendered or outright sexist comments and attitudes persist. As a result, genderedness is constantly a key ingredient for participating in school life.

Joanna Thornborrow's (2014) research highlights the ways that teachers control classroom participation through their teacher talk. She sees teacher talk as creating and maintaining asymmetrical power relationships. Teacher-led classroom talk as a pedagogical approach is often organized around initiation/ response/follow-up exchanges in which the teacher controls the students by controlling the dynamics of classroom discourse: 'the teacher takes turns at will, allocates turns to others, determines topics, interrupts and reallocates turns judged to be irrelevant to these topics, and provides a running commentary on what is being said and meant' (p. 176).

Thornborrow's conclusions complement earlier feminist ideas, such as Pat Mahony's (1985), that pointed to classrooms as sites of patriarchy. Mahony understood teacher attention swayed towards the boys as an indication of prevailing societal attitudes which stem from attitudes at large: that boys are privileged learners as males are privileged participants in society, and that this privilege is evidenced in the way boys monopolize teacher attention. In Mahony's study, for every two boys asking questions there was only one girl. Michelle Stanworth's (1983) work also explored gender divisions in classroom talk, and her conclusions also rested significantly on teacher control of classroom talk. She said:

> The important point is not that girls are being 'discriminated against', in the sense of being graded more harshly or denied educational opportunities but that the classroom is a venue in which girls and boys, dependent upon a [teacher] who has a considerable degree of power over their immediate comfort and long-term future, can hardly avoid becoming enmeshed in a process whereby 'normal' relationships between the sexes are being constantly defined. (p. 18)

Studies which have involved protracted observation of a variety of classrooms have shown, almost invariably, that boys receive a disproportionate share of teachers' time and attention. High achieving boys in some studies are a particularly favored group, claiming more of their teachers' energies than either similarly performing girls or less successful pupils of either sex. On the other hand, although girls were criticized at least as often as boys for academic mistakes, boys were far more often reprimanded for misconduct and, in some classrooms, these criticisms accounted for a large share of the extra attention directed at boys.

It has been well argued by both Mahony and Stanworth (as well as many other educational researchers in the 1980s) that the implicit message to all students was that extra time given to male students suggested to both boys and girls that boys were more interesting to the teacher. Stanworth (1983) said it like this: '...[B]y more frequently criticizing their male pupils, teachers may unwittingly reinforce the idea that the "naughtiness" of boys is more interesting, more deserving, than the "niceness" of girls' (p. 19).

If it is the case that boys receive extra attention in the classroom and that there is more dynamic talk between teachers and boys, then we must consider the issue of girls' relative silence in these same classrooms. Anthropologist Shirley Ardener's (2005) theoretical frame, Muted Group Theory, explained how it is that certain groups are 'muted' in particular contexts. American scholar, Dale Spender (1980/1990) explored the particular patterns of silence among females and reflected on the 'chattering female' stereotype as echoed in many classrooms. That is, although we perceive girls as chatty, the opposite is the case in classroom lessons where they are not very vocal. Spender said that both sexes brought to the classroom an understanding that it is the boys who should 'have the floor' and females who should be dutiful and attentive listeners. She believed that, within educational institutions, girls were made aware that their talk was evaluated differently from the boys. As such, they shut up.

Most recent research points to the underachievement of boys in part due to a growing culture of masculinity which insists on a lack of interest in academic pursuits. Lindsay and Muijs (2006), Martino (2008) and Hartley and Sutton (2013), among others, focus on masculinities in schools – on how language is used to align with a certain belonging of masculinities. The way boys speak to each other, other students and their teacher positions them in particular roles and often directs them into identities as underachievers.

However, the underachievement of boys is unlikely to benefit girls in the long run because 'discursive practices continue to constitute girls' school successes in limited and derogatory ways' (Baxter, 2003: 94). Baxter saw that even if and when girls 'win', they still 'lose'. They are 'winning' at tests but 'losing' at life. Academic successes do not correlate with senior positions in places of business later on. Even when girls overachieve at school, they opt out of career fast-tracks often because of their commitments to home and family. Regardless of which gender may be seen as 'losing out' in education (or maybe because of the confusion), gender remains a compelling variable to examine what influences academic experience. A consensus is far from imminent, and the feminist concerns that have perhaps been seen as part of a 1970s and 1980s agenda are anything but resolved even with our current preoccupation with boys' underachievement (Mahony, 1998). Regardless of who is winning at the game of educational achievement, gender matters.

It is a strong possibility, as made evident in much of the research of the 1970s and 1980s, that there has been an implicit message that girls count less to teachers, which mirrors larger social values concerning those born female. This message may well reinforce a negative self-image and lead to withdrawal from participation on the part of female students. Research has consistently suggested that boys in classrooms talk more, exert more control over talk, and interrupt other speakers more often (Coates, 1993; West & Zimmerman, 1987). Girls are assumed to listen more and to be more supportive when they do talk, largely serving as audience to a dynamic predominantly controlled by boys. Both female and male teachers tend to pay less attention to girls than to boys at all ages, in various socio-economic and ethnic groupings, and in all subjects. Girls receive less behavioral criticism, fewer instructional contacts, fewer high-level questions and academic criticism, and slightly less praise than boys across the age ranges and in all subjects (Graddol & Swann, 1989). Also, some reports found that teachers direct more open-ended questions at boys in the early years of schooling, and more yes/no questions at girls (Fichtelius *et al.*, 1980). It also appears that boys tend to be 'first in' to classroom discussions because of the teachers' own non-verbal cues, particularly their 'gaze-attention', and that this eye contact is important in systematically offering boys more opportunities for participation (Jule, 2004; Paechter, 1998; Swann, 1988, 1992, 1998).

Girls may be systematically marginalized in general class discussions and, likewise, boys seem to be given more attention by their teachers and their school communities more consistently. Arguably, such marginalization denies girls the opportunity to work through their ideas with language or to practice and experiment with spoken language. As such, there is a systemic and stubborn perpetuation of genderedness.

Speaking About Sex

Rosemary Westwood (2016), Canadian journalist, writes about the changing roles of teenagers' sexuality as a central aspect of their discourse with the opposite sex, including her observation of how quickly this change in roles is occurring. She says,

> I never got this message: 'SEND NOODZ'. That text marks the beginning of a deeply upsetting foray into the world's [...] teenager. (p. 10)

She goes on to highlight the ways social media have changed teenage life. In particular, she says, 'Digital pornography is catching children at their sexual awakening' (p. 10). As such, the way schools deal with sexual health education is now incredibly explicit – much more than it has been historically. The changing nature of the sex health curriculum requires teachers, administrators and parents to work together on how best to 'talk' about sex within the context of today's children and young adults.

Certainly the situation for girls is a 'complicated landscape', according to Erin Anderson (in Orenstein, 2016). Psychologists Zimbardo and Coulombe's (2016) new book, *Man Interrupted*, outlines disturbing statistics of the amount of pornography the average 15-year-old boy watches. The average teenage boy has had 1,400 pornographic encounters before his first actual sexual encounter with a partner. Zimbardo fears that such over-exposure to pornography (along with excessive video gaming and/or drugs and alcohol) creates 'moodles' (man poodles) who are unable to engage in real relationships or care for themselves and, thus, remain stunted throughout their lives. How do schools and classroom teachers deal with such a context?

For one, it is important to understand that reliance on pornography undermines normal sexual development. With pornography, the ups and downs of a real relationship are absent, turning sex into nothing more than a physical activity. If desire emerges through pornography, it can take away desire from real sex with real people. When individuals steeped in the world of pornography enter the 'real world', they flounder. As such, many sexual health educators believe it is necessary to speak directly about the effects of pornography in any sex education curriculum.

The over-saturation of sex in today's youth culture has taken its toll. In her 2016 book, *Talk Sex Today*, Canadian sexual-health educator, Saleema Noon, relates this anecdote about a 15-year-old boy:

> At a house party, a girl he barely knew offered to give him oral sex in a back bedroom. 'Nah, I'm good,' he told her. He 'made the mistake' of telling his friends, who called him a 'wuss' and a 'fag' for turning down a 'hot chick'.

In light of such realities, it seems clear that, while girls experience *slut-shaming*, boys experience equally troubling demands by peers: many teens do experience their sexuality in relation to their peers. To interrupt a steady stream of sexual imagery and experimentalism will take a kind of 'direct talk' on the part of the teacher. But this in and of itself can be difficult. Education systems have always struggled with how to handle emerging sexuality in schools; with such a sex-saturated culture, it makes things even more difficult.

In contemporary Western societies, there is phenomenal and rapid change regarding gender relations in general. There are extraordinary contradictions and constructions of gender in the media. For example, Rosalind Gill (2007) mentions the rise of 'girl power' that sits alongside reports of 'epidemic' levels of anorexia and body dysmorphia. While some aspects of feminism go unmarked, other aspects of feminism face more bitter repudiation than at any other time in history. One wonders if the more powerful women become, the greater the desire is to diminish them? Is it possible that the extraordinary proliferation of discourse about sex and sexuality, including the 'increasingly frequent erotic presentation of girls' (Gill, 2007), has led to the sexualization of culture itself? Such questions are important to explore within any effective sex education program. The rise of 'porn culture' and the necessary misogyny that creates it is witnessed in such places as Reddit, music videos, and on TV, in the vitriolic attacks on women who fail to live up to increasingly narrow requirements.

Reporting Sexual Violence on Campus

It is now estimated that between 20 and 25% of college/university women either have been raped, or attempts have been made to rape them over the course of their college years. In most cases (9 out of 10), the victims of rape knew their offender as many of the rapes or attempted rapes happen during a date. For every 1,000 women attending a college or university, there are 35 incidents of rape of university students, with 66% happening off campus. And yet, less than 5% of completed rapes are ever reported to the police or to school officials.

Most young women will confide in a close friend but rarely report to officials or even to family members (Fisher *et al.*, 2000). The numbers are remarkably consistent across all Western countries. Researchers have been looking for patterns to this trend, finding that most sexual assaults occur in September, October and November, and on Friday and Saturday nights between the hours of midnight and 6am (Krebs *et al.*, 2007). Some reports suggest alcohol plays a key role in the rape culture, particularly on campuses where binge-drinking is high (Mohler-Kuo *et al.*, 2004). Alcohol and substance abuse appear to be linked to unsafe and abusive sexual practices, and it is young female students new to campus life who are most vulnerable. But why do young women (and others) report rape so rarely?

Educational institutes are places where society itself seeks to reproduce the status quo. As such, the persistent rates of sexual assault at universities is highly problematic and says much about society's view of women. The systemic misogyny which surrounds this issue is key. Many feminist scholars see the 'unequal and coercive practices' as made 'common in heterosexual relationships' underlying the necessity of understanding these relationships that come through power inequalities. These practices intersect in complex and sometimes contradictory ways with other forms of inequality on campus – in particular, class, age and geographical origin (Clowes *et al.*, 2008: 30). A disregard for the honor of others seems endemic in all societies, and schools are not only not immune to these realities, they are often sites of the reproduction of related attitudes and behaviors.

Young women are likely hesitant to report rape because of the response when they do. They are often not believed or accused of encouraging rape by what they have worn or where they were or how much they were drinking or if they were involved in drug use. But the objective fact is that young women get raped because someone rapes them. Even in high-profile sexual assault cases, the victims become victims again to the attitudes of society at large suspicious of young women's version of events.

A now-famous case of 'Jackie' reported in *Rolling Stone* magazine of an alleged 2012 rape by members of a fraternity turned out to be entirely fabricated. But the article made a strong point concerning the lived reality for young women who are victims of sexual assault and are then met with doubt and resistance from so-called friends and administrators. Few forgave *Rolling Stone* for publishing the fictionalized story as if true, claiming their reasons for having written it were simply for shock value. In fact, some feminists were furious that the eventual retraction strengthened the argument that women lie about sexual assaults, noting that it 'heightened the belief that women lie' (Stoddard, 2015). Needless to say, the fraternity in question and a number of university alumni sued *Rolling Stone*.

Sable *et al.* (2006) asked college students to rate the importance of a list of barriers in reporting rape and sexual assault among both male and female victims, including shame, guilt, embarrassment, not wanting friends and family to know, concerns about confidentiality, and fear of not being believed. Both genders perceived a fear of being judged as 'gay' to be an important barrier for male victims of sexual assault or rape and fear of retaliation by the perpetrator a strong barrier for female victims. The hesitation for reporting rape is embedded in community and cultural norms, thus demonstrating the need for community-focused solutions.

Silence as Participation Strategy

Silence among many female students seems to be a comfortable participation strategy used by those born female because more verbal interaction by girls in classrooms is often condemned as 'chatty' and 'trivial'. Of particular concern to many feminists is the connection between gender, speech and silence – what Pat Mahony (1985) termed 'linguistic space'. Mahony found that it was 'normal' for a teacher to ignore girls for long periods of time, for boys to call out, and for boys to dominate classroom talk in addition to dominating the actual physical space. This evidence of gendered language tendencies regarding the use of linguistic space in classrooms may derive from both the particular features of the language used (specific patterns and habits of belonging) as well as the amount or proportion of talk-time in teacher-led lessons. That is, it is both the quality of language as well as the quantity that seem to reinforce gender divisions.

Gender roles are constructed through language, and teachers in particular pass on the social order through their own use of speech, including the proportions of talk-time and the level of meaningful discussions. Such 'gendering' may be seen most obviously in the proportion of talk-time. Mahony's (1985) evidence was that a disproportionate amount of linguistic space is allotted to males in classrooms and this has an effect on the female classroom experience.

Even if or when the attention paid to boys is negative, their very presence in the classroom claims more teacher time and focus (Paechter, 1998). Teachers' attempts to get boys to consent to their authority might be one reason they allow boys more control over physical space, teacher attention and lesson content. But with the importance of student-centred learning in today's schools, classroom talk is becoming increasingly seen as central to the learning process. The range of international research has persuasively demonstrated that the skill to speak effectively in public confers social and/ or professional prestige, and that this usually falls to the males in any given society (Baxter, 2003; Coates, 1993; Holmes, 1998; Jones & Mahony, 1989; Nichols, 1998; Tannen, 1995). Speaking up in class is not just important for the opportunity to engage with ideas or with the language: it signifies and creates important social power and legitimacy. Hence, educators and educational institutions should have the obligation to be aware of the performance of gender.

Relationships within classrooms may well propel the gender imbalance that is seen in society more generally. The implications of the gender imbalance point to the possibility of girls having less opportunity to speak aloud or publicly engage with ideas. This loss of opportunity may result in girls' lower confidence and their receiving less recognition or encouragement when they do speak aloud. In the rapid exchange in classroom discussions of teacher-student talk, it is often the first student who responds by raising a hand or making eye contact with the teacher who receives the attention of the class. Swann (1998) and many others have suggested that such quick responders are usually male. By engaging in a form of privileged interaction, teachers are not only distancing those who may be less competitive or aggressive, but are also giving those who already excel in claiming the floor (often the boys) further opportunities to do so.

If girls and boys tend to have markedly different patterns in their use of language in many classrooms and across various age groups, then these patterns may reflect the language patterns around them, as well as develop these patterns further. If teaching methods offer little recognition of the possibility of gendered language experiences and create unequal language opportunities for the students as a result, if there is a marked gender difference in the use of linguistic space, then this needs to be further examined by researchers and classroom teachers alike.

In Lakoff's (1975) seminal work, she called for a 'relearning of language' that would require those born female to recognize those speech patterns that undermine power, throw off their 'learned helplessness', and simply speak more 'like men'. However, when applied to classroom life in particular, there is no empirical evidence to suggest that if girls used more interruptions, for example, that this would dismantle patriarchy and create greater female power – for them or females in general. The day-to-day experiences are too complicated for such simplistic self-help directives. Nevertheless, awareness of gendered tendencies in classroom talk is an important step in seeking gender parity and in seeing how it is that gender roles and behaviors are socialized by environment.

However, silence may or may not be a conscious strategy on the part of females. Coates (1993) identifies silence as part of her discussion of the societal perception of female 'verbosity' and the cultural requirement for females to say less. She cites Soskin and John's early (1963) study that found it was men who took longer to describe a picture (average 13 minutes) as compared to women (average three minutes); and that males usually took up to four times the *linguistic space* in most circumstances. Coates suggests that the myth of females as talkative leads to certain expectations of who has the right to talk. Here she agrees with Spender's (1980) hypothesis that female speech is often viewed as empty 'chatter' and trivial, while what men say is viewed as important and significant.

As seems clear to me, much research has been carried out in classrooms in a search for the nature and underlying basis for gendered speech and has highlighted distinct gendered expectations. Much has been found to solidify the claim that females and males in classrooms use – or are allowed to use – language differently, have differing motivations to do so, and that their speech is interpreted differently even if they use the same speech strategies (Hall & Bucholtz, 1995; Talbot, 1998; Wodak, 1997). The examination of male/female differences in classroom interactions may be complicated by context, power and interpretation of the very same linguistic forms when aligned with sex. Nonetheless, certainly some differences appear with regularity across cultures and across social groups and highlight classrooms as key sites for gender rehearsal.

Summing Up

- Gender roles and expectations are prescribed early in life and are accepted and rehearsed by very young children in the school system as stable characteristics.
- Teachers are often unaware of the ways boys and girls are treated in the classroom, believing they 'treat them all the same' when, in fact, boys and girls are responded to in differing ways throughout the school years.
- Silence among many female students seems to be a comfortable participation strategy used by those born female because more verbal interaction by girls in classrooms is often condemned as 'chatty' and 'trivial'.

5

Gender and Language Use in the Workplace

. . . .

We need to reshape our own perception of how we view ourselves.
We have to step up as women and take the lead.

Beyoncé

Research from the 1970s to the 1990s examining language and gender in the workplace was heavily influenced by popular paradigms at the time, namely the deficit and dominance approaches. As women began to enter the workplace in greater numbers throughout the 20th century, language and gender research in this area started to grow, and a number of key studies were produced. The early studies took gender difference as a given. Some tended to focus on the domain of medicine, particularly doctor–patient interactions (West, 1984, 1990). Bonnie McElhinny (1998) explored women police officers; William O'Barr and Bowman Atkins (1998) looked at women in courts of law; and others explored women in politics, in broadcast journalism, at church, in school leadership and even in hairdressing. According to these studies, the power that more men have over more women in society is reflected in many workplace encounters.

Framing Gender in Workplace Relationships

The research examines the linguistic strategies that women and men adopt in both single- and mixed-sex workplace settings. Certainly by the mid-1990s, social constructionist approaches to language and gender began to develop and take root. In addition to the notion of 'doing gender' in various 'communities of practice', some, such as Shari Kendall and Deborah Tannen (1997), drew on the notion of 'framing' as helpful in understanding various interactions. Women and men often 'frame' themselves based on societal gendered norms for appropriate behavior and their own self-concept. Kendall and Tannen argued that the relationship between language and gender was 'sex-class' linked; that is, spoken interaction was not necessarily identified with a woman or man but was rather associated with 'women as a class' or 'men as a class' within society. They saw that individuals align themselves with a particular sex-class by talking in a particular way that is associated with that sex-class: they frame themselves.

Discursive and social constructionist approaches have been particularly important in workplace studies. Studies by Janet Holmes and her colleagues are good examples of such approaches. In 1996, Holmes set up a government-funded project in Wellington, New Zealand, entitled *Language and the Workplace*. Early publications associated with this project demonstrate the transition in language and gender studies away from the dominance and difference paradigms of the 1970s and 1980s and towards the more dynamic 'communities of practice' social constructionist approaches (Holmes, 2000a; Holmes *et al.*, 2001). Holmes's work is important because it suggests it is not possible to make generalizations about the behavior of 'women' versus 'men' at work. There are myriad complexities, particular roles, professional identities and social contexts that influence each interaction.

While there may be some evidence of gendered patterning, there is also more and more compelling evidence that while gendered interactional styles may be stereotypically 'true', they are in no way universal. To say that there is a feminine style of leadership and to say that it is indirect, conciliatory, facilitative or collaborative, while a masculine style is more direct, aggressive, competitive and autonomous is overtly sexist as well as inaccurate. Holmes's analysis of the speech strategies of successful women managers in positions of power found that they were using a 'wide-verbal-repertoire style' (Holmes, 2000a: 13). All the women managers Holmes examined were evaluated as being effective by their colleagues, regardless of their sex. Holmes attributes workplace success to a mixture of stereotypical masculine and feminine discourse styles that women managers in her study used to achieve their goals. While Holmes did not look at men as managers, others have. Case (1995) argued that a full repertoire of styles with men and women displaying characteristics stereotypically associated with masculine and feminine speech, enables participants to be simultaneously assertive and supportive. That is, both styles are effective for both sexes in particular contexts. It is not an 'either/or' but a 'both/and'.

Chipping Away at the Glass Ceiling

In the last year or so, we saw this study, from America, and it broke our hearts a bit, because it explains so much: in a mixed-gender group, when women talk 25% of the time or less, it's seen as being 'equally balanced'. And if women talk 25–50% of the time, they're seen as 'dominating the conversation' – making some sense of the 'women are everywhere' sentiment. If there are more than one quarter it's too much. (Moran, 2011)

This quote is by Caitlin Moran, author of *How to be a Woman*, who participated in *Esquire* magazine's special 'women and men' section in the March 2016 issue. The issue also featured a conversation on gender relations with Hollywood actor Tom Hanks and the young British actor Emma Watson, whose initiative as a UN Women Global Goodwill Ambassador, *HeForShe*, has been devoted to uniting men and women in the goal of gender parity.

Regardless of the ways men and women have been framed by gendered identities, and regardless of the use of both masculine and feminine styles in successful leaders in the workplace, it remains the case that more men succeed in the traditional world of business and workplace settings. That women cannot achieve top levels of leadership is known as *the glass ceiling* – an invisible force that keeps women from succeeding to levels that men can in a particular profession.

The glass ceiling is primarily about two things: visibility and power, and not separately but in combination. It seems to be the case that, in spite of the many feminist advances concerning education and gender equity laws, there are fewer women who have access to real power or who exercise visible power in the workplace. It seems fine for women to be visible in various places of business as long as they don't have any meaningful or serious power. There are plenty of women who serve as vice-presidents or vice-principals but fewer who are presidents of major companies or heads of major educational institutions. That is to say, women are in important jobs, but they usually answer to a man at the top of the chain. It seems okay for women to have power, as long as they are behind the scenes or not exercising that power too visibly. This discrepancy is seen in countries around the world. Though this is quickly changing, in 2000 in the United States, women comprised 46.5% of the American workforce but held only 12% of upper management level positions (Wichterich, 2000).

There has been a tendency since the 1960s both in business and in other industries to consider the issue of civil rights and gender parity. It has only been about 40 years since women have been easily promoted and invited into roles of leadership. Even so, it seems that no matter how competent, well-educated or successful she is, a woman can only go so far. The existence of some success stories does not eliminate the fact that in many professional circumstances, the workplace is not a level playing field for most women. Globally, women who have graduated from university are paid 18% less than their male counterparts. In banking, insurance, and pension programs, women earn 70 cents for every dollar a man earns. Female academics earn $10,000 (USD) less per year than their male colleagues (Wichterich, 2000).

It is my view that the turning back or dropping out that occurs when women hit the glass ceiling has a direct and devastating effect on the work-place. To not have women in various kinds of employment, including top positions of leadership, means that aspiring men and women cannot see that success can be genderless. Without a balance, leadership can feel contrived and manipulated. Entire communities are profoundly negatively affected when role models do achieve but are then treated unjustly in some way. The lack of women in both real and visible positions of power is more than a token of fairness; it restricts women from being fully human and from encountering a wide variety of experiences and, maybe more importantly, society is diminished by the absence of many voices.

Clearly, blocking women from fully participating in society violates basic human rights. It is important to consider why some women are excluded – why do so many women around the world hit the 'glass ceiling' in various career paths? What are some factors that work against women in senior positions in a variety of employment situations? Certainly the use of language is a key factor.

The ultimate glass ceiling is the top political position of power – leading a country. Though countries in Africa and Asia have had female leaders at the top, the position of women in politics in the West reveals a painful, stubborn and confusing relationship with women on top. Such women are suspect for having the ambition for such positions and then must deal with consistent attacks on their womanhood, including their role as mother (or not) and/or as a wife. Their leadership qualities appear as only one aspect of them while their capacities in their personal lives are fodder for the press. The lives of Angela Merkel of Germany, Theresa May of Great Britain, Nicola Sturgeon of Scotland and Hillary Clinton in the US are under constant surveillance. Clinton's loss of the presidential election in 2016 is a prime example of how vicious politics in the West can be for women – even at the hands of other women. [Note: White, evangelical women did not vote for Hillary.] Another example of this was seen in the summer of 2016 when the Brexit vote in the UK brought a crisis of leadership. The then Prime Minister, David Cameron, resigned immediately following the vote, leaving the Conservative party to choose a new leader. When the decision was between two women, one of them (Andrea Leadsom) suggested her role as mother gave her the advantage for the job as Prime Minister, over the childless (or childfree) Theresa May (Elgot, 2016).

In 2012, former Australian Prime Minister Julia Gillard stood up in Parliament to charge the current Prime Minister as a misogynist. The YouTube clip of her 'misogyny speech' went viral even while the all-male Australian press gallery shrugged it off. It appeared that her speech touched a nerve; Gillard voiced the words that many women would want to say about the misogynistic work environments in which they live their lives (Keneally, 2015). Recently, a local Member of the Legislative Assembly in the Canadian province of Alberta, Sandra Jansen, stood up in the legislature and read aloud sexist/abusive messages she has received while in office, including words like 'bitch', 'dumb broad' and 'bimbo' (Anderson, 2016). In that case, the entire Alberta legislature rose to its feet with applause of support for her motion to ban sexism from government business. Even when the glass ceiling is broken, women in positions of power are still subject to double standards and intense personal judgement.

Gender at Work

Today's young women rank among the most educated in history, yet many also grapple with frustrations never imagined by their mothers or grandmothers. Canadian researcher Lesley Andres (2004) gathered 15 years of data on Canadian youth's transition to adulthood. She studied 700 women and men from 1988 to 2003 as they moved their way through early adulthood and into middle age. Andres's work suggests that Canadian women, despite having earned comparable post-secondary credentials, are twice as likely as men to be employed part-time, and tend to pool in the clerical, sales and services sector. In contrast, men work primarily in middle management and as semi-professionals or professionals. Andres points out that it can take a woman 15 years (on average) to catch up with men in the area of employer-paid benefits if she has children. Andres suggests that it is the educational choices of teenaged boys that are the most relevant; that is, highly educated boys have consistently the most successful career trajectories over highly educated girls who often 'opt-out' of a career path to bear and tend children at a critical stage in career development.

Male stereotyping and preconceptions of women are two of the biggest barriers women face at work; while these fences do not necessarily point to blatant sexism, they are indicators of people espousing outdated ideas rooted in stereotypes about women's abilities and commitment to their careers. Other obstacles include exclusion from informal networks of communication (like the golf club) and a lack of mentors. Women often feel excluded from casual situations and social settings (having drinks, going for lunch) where deals are discussed, and female mentors are few. A senior man seems more likely to take a younger man under his wing and introduce him to important people. Women, however, are often left to navigate the political waters of any given organization on their own. Many women need to 'opt out' even when they have opportunities because of the lifestyle decisions that are necessary in achieving and holding positions of power and come at great personal cost (www.womensmedia. com, 2003).

Research in the public and private sectors also suggests that at least 50% of women have experienced sexual harassment at work. Sexual harassment can take many forms, including propositions, jokes, suggestive comments, innuendo and comments about appearance. It also seems to be a vicious circle: women experience more frustration and exclusion in positions of leadership, so they 'opt-out', and then fewer of them are there to mentor and guide others. Also, their opting-out may serve as evidence that women can't (or won't) handle it.

Lean In: Gender and Styles of Leadership

'Women at work' is a complicated issue because, in society, women and men are not set up to be all that comfortable working with each other. There are often feelings of confusion, irritation and discomfort between the sexes because of the lack of experience together and the rehearsal in different gender cultures that occurs throughout our lives. Women seem to be associated with certain attributes, like the ability to share power and information, to multi-task and to build consensus. These are positive traits regardless of one's sex. Even so, men are often selected for top jobs based on perceived potential rather than actual performance and/or because their leadership style is seen as more authoritative, more commanding and more confident. Working together can be uncomfortable, and discomfort feeds frustration for both men and women.

Some studies have attempted to articulate some genderedness in the workplace. For example, the early work of Mintzberg (1973) found that men in business tended to:

1. work at an unrelenting pace, with no breaks in activity during the day
2. stop when there is an interruption, discontinuity and fragmentation
3. spare little time for activities not directly related to their work
4. establish a preference for live action encounters
5. maintain a complex network of relationships with people outside of their organization (peers, colleagues, clients for the purposes of information gathering)
6. immersing themselves in the day-to-day need to keep the company going, they lack time for reflection
7. identify themselves with their jobs (strong identity to job role)
8. have difficulty sharing information (information as power and they are reluctant to share the information, causing overburdened workloads because the decisions always required them)

Sally Helgesen (1995) revisited Mintzberg's study and attempted to examine women's style of leadership. She found that women tended to:

1. work at a steady pace, but with small breaks throughout the day (used the breaks for returning phone calls or following up on tasks)
2. not view unscheduled tasks and encounters as interruptions but as key to the working of the business (women used words like caring, being involved, helping and being responsible)
3. take time for activities not directly related to their work
4. prefer live action encounters, but schedule time to attend to mail
5. maintain a complex network of relationships with people outside their organizations
6. focus on the ecology of leadership (keep to a long-term focus)
7. see their own identities as complex and multi-faceted
8. schedule in time for sharing information

Regardless of sex, however, definitions of gendered leadership can be distracting as well as incredibly inaccurate. What is worth considering is the demands on those in leadership positions and the unrelenting pressures in capitalist societies for a certain demand for success. This drive for personal success can limit both men's and women's connection to their families and communities. In any event, both men and women can display a variety of leadership attributes and styles that cross gender stereotypes. Surely both 'masculine' and 'feminine' styles have an important part to play in workplace success.

Louise Mullany (2003) examined gendered discourses in interviews with female and male managers at middle and senior managerial levels in Britain. One of her aims was to discuss participants' managerial roles and the impact of gender on their everyday work lives. The results suggested that women in positions of authority are often evaluated negatively, even in spite of their success in their jobs. Mullany suggests that this is in large part due to the ideal of femininity that centers around physical appearance rather than competence. Only when women look the 'right' way for the job are they viewed positively. The women themselves were very aware of this as the requirement for success, and they felt trapped by it. The view perpetuated by the dominant discourse of femininity regarding the feminine image appears to be that women need to be slim, attractive and well-groomed to be taken seriously in the workplace.

The discourse of female emotionality also plays a part in the gender in the workplace conversation. Mullany's interviews record men articulating stereotypical views about that 'one week a month' when women are more emotional and therefore incapable of being rational at work. Others, such as Lazar (2005), have argued that gender in the workplace reveals a deeply embedded androcentrism in which both men and women are complicit. Even if professionals see the skills of men and women as interchangeable in positions at work, there is a perception that it is based entirely on the individual's ability for success (or not) and not reliant on social forces – that individuality is the main cause of success or failure. It seems that gender can be used as an excuse for some and viewed as a non-issue by others.

Mansplaining is a term used to identify a manner of speaking where someone (typically a man) explains something to someone else (typically a woman) in a condescending or patronizing manner. Women at work face patronizing 'explaination' by some men at work regardless of any power difference. Even the Premier of British Columbia in Canada complained about 'mansplaining' in her role dealing with men, assuming she must be unaware of all necessary information and feeling obliged to inform her (Clark, 2016).

When former President Obama took office in 2008, two-thirds of his top aides were men. Women complained. They began speaking out about having to 'elbow their way in to important meetings' and how their voices were often ignored even when they managed to get in. These female staffers 'adopted a meeting strategy'. If a woman made a point during a meeting, another woman would repeat it and say aloud the woman's name, such as 'Peggy makes an excellent point'. They saw how this strategy forced the men in the room to pay attention to women's contributions and to keep men from claiming the ideas as their own (Eilperin, 2016). They call this strategy 'amplification'.

Perhaps it is no surprise that academic scholars would turn the lens on their own workplaces. British, American, Australian and Canadian universities cite similar trends of more women academics entering the profession. However, women's jobs in academia tend to be more junior, more teaching-based, more pastoral, and often part-time.

Sally McConnell-Ginet (2000) wonders if, when achievement is rewarded, men get credit for determination and commitment, while women are seen as lucky and having to work extraordinarily hard to fulfill the task. Claire Walsh (2001) found that women's increased presence in traditionally male-dominated workplaces such as academia has resulted in a 'strengthening of fraternal networks' and a blocking out of women. Also, Barbara Reskin and Patricia Roos (1990) claim that women typically enter fields that men no longer find desirable due to loss of pay, prestige or autonomy. This possibility may help to explain women in junior positions within academia – men don't want the extra burden of teaching positions, so women can have them. Such explanations may also help explain the increase of women in the medical profession and in the clergy over the last 30 years. Alternatively, Reskin and Roos see men entering certain jobs once viewed as only for women, like nursing, as raising the status of the job.

Whether women are fluent in cooperative styles or not, researchers like Lia Litosseliti (2006) see that assumptions about gender positions are powerful. Especially in male-dominated workplaces – business organizations, government, politics, the church, the police, the law – where assertive behavior is necessary, women must constantly negotiate gender assumptions and expectations. For example, Bonnie McElhinny (2003) explores how women police officers tend to 'masculinize' their behavior and refrain from cooperative strategies in order to be effective.

According to Litosseliti, the appropriation of 'masculine' styles by women in such communities is understandable, given the historical context of struggle for women to gain access to certain roles. Because of this, Litosseliti believes that women often adopt interactional approaches that align with leadership styles. Judith Baxter's (2006) collection of research on the female voice in public contexts provides insight on how women both appropriate masculine public discourse and find new ways of combining 'doing leadership' and 'doing gender' successfully.

It is also possible that, with time, we will become increasingly comfortable working with both sexes in various workplace settings and this in and of itself will alter stereotypes. This comfort can come with time, experience and effort. However, if women are squeezed out of positions of leadership and allocated to the three Cs (childcare, cleaning and clerical roles), then we deny the gifts embedded in each person. If men are denied lives more concerned with family and personal pursuits, then we deny them fuller, more meaningful lives. Likewise, if women are denied access to top levels of leadership, then we deny them fuller, more meaningful lives as well.

Summing Up

- Most positions of influence in our society (such as medicine, law, politics, business) attract men who are trained to lead and are more comfortable in positions requiring authority and certainty.
- Even while today's women are the most educated in history, many opt-out of top positions because of the impossible demands of both the workplace and their private lives.
- The glass ceiling does not signify just a personal loss for some women; it also influences society by removing women from visibility and from power. This has negative consequences for both women and men by limiting our human connections.

6

Gender and Language Use in Religion: Judaism, Christianity and Islam

. . . .

Feminism's agenda is basic: It asks that women not be
forced to 'choose' between public justice and private happiness.

Susan Faludi

All societies fumble with ever-changing gender roles and identities; the complexities of globalization and multiculturalism intersect to influence the pace and the extent of changes. Religions across the world attempt, in various ways, to respond to various gender and sexuality issues of modern life in the 21st century. This includes religious communities. What interests me about the connection of gender and language use alongside religion is the significance of words to belief – and the significance of discourse in revealing certain religious beliefs. Even while the West experiences increased *secularization*, religious communities continue to gain in popularity worldwide. I grew up in the Catholic faith and attended Catholic schools. I believe my experiences with a traditional religious community have influenced my genderedness and my connection to religious discourse as a way of belonging to corporate worship (like the Mass). This chapter considers some general ways that language and gender have connected with religion.

In today's global pluralism, almost any faith can be found anywhere, as a secure and steady presence for some and as a personal option or expression regarding religious persuasion for others. Hinduism, Buddhism and Islam (religions originating in the East) are found all over the West, and the various representations of the West's Judaism and Christianity are now well established throughout the world. The massive rise in American-style politically right-wing evangelical Christianity has been a fascinating sociological phenomenon for some time – both in the US and in other countries around the world – as has radical fundamentalist Islam. Religion and religious groups influence the geopolitical world in regards to war zones, political campaigns and world governance. The rise of ISIS: the (so-called) Islamic State, a terrorist organization who claim to emerge from Islam, has massively influenced world events and shifts in geopolitical alliances. As such, the connections of gender and language with particular religious expressions make for fascinating case studies.

Gender in the World Religions

The majority of the world's population today regard themselves as religious in one way or another. The growing numbers might surprise those who are familiar with the influential secular ideology of the West. A 2008 Gallup poll asked people in over 140 countries whether religion was an important part of their lives; 82% said yes (Mezit, 2011: 21).

Because gender is socially constructed, it is fascinating to see how gender roles, expectations, and behaviors play out in religious communities. It is of 'great significance for those who want to keep a status quo in a certain social system to insist on existing practices, values and orders. [...] Often religious institutions undertake this task' (Mezit, 2011: 4). Despite the intricate relatedness between religion and feminism (in particular, that early feminists relied on moral reasoning regarding the equality of all people as central to the Christian faith), many religious people discard feminism because they associate it with a secular worldview. Likewise, many feminists discard religion as a matter of course because of the deep patriarchy at the core of religious dogma.

Judith Plaskow (1990), in her feminist book *Standing Again at Sinai*, discusses and criticizes the either/or attitudes among her religious community – Judaism. She says that she is 'particularly annoyed by the fact that the majority of Jewish women never question aspects of Judaism' (p. x) that are, according to her, misogynistic. The same kind of reluctance to identify with feminism is seen across Christian and Muslim communities as well. In particular, many devout Muslims reject feminism on the grounds that it is an idea that has come from the West, and they view such ideas of equality for women as products of Western neo-imperialism (Mezit, 2011). Others claim that both Christianity and Islam recognized the equality of women over a thousand years ago. Some members of all three of these faiths see the notion of perceiving God (or Allah) as male to be deeply problematic, since viewing God as male necessitates viewing what is male as more divine than what is female. Christian feminists point to the feminist and egalitarian attitude of Christ and positive female imagery in the Bible. Islamic feminists also see the Qur'an as egalitarian and want re-readings of patriarchal texts and rules that they believe male-dominated hierarchies have erased.

Based on the creation account in the Torah, the Bible and the Qur'an, some religious communities justify religious misogyny based on the following:

- Man was created first, hence he is superior to woman.
- The purpose of woman's creation was to help man and give him company.
- Woman is derived from man.
- Woman is easily tempted.
- God has cursed women with pain in childbearing. (Mezit, 2011: 39)

This list is relevant to all three major monotheistic faiths. For Jewish, Christian and Muslim feminists, these interpretations of the key creation story reveal the social attitudes at the time by the authors who wrote them – men.

Islam is the most controversial religion today. Lejla Mezit (2011) explains some of the most significant issues within the discourse on Islam and gender: wife-beating, female legal inferiority, marital rape, polygamy, female circumcision, forced marriages and hijab (the Islamic dress code). Yet she also questions why it is that these issues make the front pages while misogyny in Judaism and Christianity receive less media attention – and by extension appear to be less political. In any case, the sacred texts on which the three major monotheistic religions are based are believed by adherents to be the authentic word of God; the interpretations of these texts have changed throughout history and will likely continue to do so.

A good example of the vicissitudes and rifts within major religions can be found in the story of the Canadian Anglican bishop Michael Ingham who, in 2007, called for a 'new theology of human sexuality' (Valpy, 2007: A3). He told a large church conference that the Christian Church's opposition to birth control, abortion, masturbation and homosexuality has been 'morally groundless'. He cited embedded patriarchy in the Church as a 'distortion of the gospel'. Other Christians disagreed, calling his remarks 'whimsical' and reckless. In such ways, the issue of gender and sex alongside religion is contentious. Angela McRobbie (1994) suggested that 'the Church [exists] alongside the pressure groups, the charities, and the voluntary organizations which, when taken as a whole, represent a strong body of public opinion' (p. 112). This is particularly evident in the US where there are now at least 70 million evangelical Christians making this particular expression the most popular religious subgroup in the Western world (Meyerhof, 2006).

Talking of God as Male

Within Christianity, much of the debate on the role of women, for example, has involved the creating of a new vision of language use, including traditional hymns and the Bible itself. Keeping in mind the patriarchal culture in which the Bible emerged some 2,000 years ago, some of today's feminist scholars have searched for and found passages and images supportive of an equal position for women. They hold the egalitarian view that female oppression in the church has been a reflection of a misogynist culture, not at all connected to holiness or godliness. They focus on the Bible's teaching that all of humanity is created equal in God's image. Feminist scholars have also offered new ways to understand some apparently patriarchal passages. Because they understand 'God' to be acting in both 'masculine' and 'feminine' ways, it is then possible to conceive of God as an entity who is beyond sex. Egalitarians hold to this view, but traditionalists/*complementarians* do not. They see gender hierarchy as part of 'God's order' of things, viewing women as created to support men.

Radical feminist and theologian Mary Daly (1973) believed that the reference to God as 'Our Father' had been disastrous – a product of human imagination that limits women's ability to fully contribute to the world around them. Deborah Cameron (1990) also attacked women's exclusion from full participation in church life, saying 'it is not just that women do not speak: often they are explicitly *prevented* from speaking, either by social taboos and restrictions or by the more genteel tyrannies of custom and practice' (p. 4).

It is no secret that male scholars have had a monopoly on most organized religions (such as Judaism, Islam, Hinduism, Buddhism and Sikhism). But once women entered the field of theology in the 1970s in particular, they were in positions to promote other scriptures that declare the equality of both men and women. Claire Walsh (2001) points to the use of certain scriptural passages over others in any religion as a 'site of ideological struggle, with a complex set of competing readings becoming polarized along gender lines' (p. 167). There are basically two views of gender and religious life: traditionalists (complementarians) and progressives (who are mainly egalitarians as regards gender). Both sides of the gender and inclusion debate see their interpretation as essential to their faith. Women are either as central as men or they have different gender roles to play.

The strength of the understanding of the male as central within many traditional faiths is most evident in the belief of an unbroken male line from Moses, Jesus or Mohammed. For some Christians (Catholics in particular), a male priest stands in for Christ: the maleness of the priest is not incidental, but theologically essential. In Islam, the issue of direct lineage with Mohammed sets up the tensions between Shia and Sunni traditions.

Mary Daly herself ultimately left her Christian community because of her view of religion as patriarchal, declaring, 'Since God is male, then the male *is* God'. According to her analysis, religious communities are locations of, and even a defense for, patriarchy. Some of the religiously devoted stay out of the debate entirely because of what they see to be more pressing social concerns such as poverty, the environment and domestic abuse. Certainly Pope Francis has been functioning as a reformer, regarding a generous inclusion of people in the Catholic Church. Many feminist theologians, like Rebecca Chopp (1989), believe that the rise in women's power is related to the diminished standing of the Church in the West. She suggests that giving more space to women in various religions has led to the rise of secularization. One of the most observable influences of feminism on Christianity in the last 30 years, for instance, is the increased number of women in positions of leadership within the Church. However, many women clergy express their frustrations with their roles and their lack of legitimacy. Being male still equates with public displays of faith and influence, while being female continues to equate with a more private, supportive expression of faithfulness (Connell, 1995; Gilligan, 1982). For religious women, they cannot veer too far off the feminine behaviors of gentleness, nurturing and thoughtfulness, even if they do hold positions of leadership, since these traits are seen as feminine ideals.

Like many egalitarian campaigners for women's ordination within the Christian church, Monica Furlong (1991) saw the campaign to have the acceptance of gender-inclusive language, such as the use of 's/he' rather than the so-called generic 'he', and 'people' rather than 'man', as central to the feminist project of securing equality for men and women within religious communities. A change of language could change the attitudes concerning women, but there have been objections. Some see inclusive language as problematic because it leads to a 'lack of dignity', a 'weakening of sense', and 'a diluting of the richness' in ancient scriptures and hymns (Thomas, 1996: 168).

Gender-neutral Language

Gender-neutral language is a style of writing and speaking that adheres to certain 'rules' that were first proposed by feminists in the 1970s. These rules prohibit common usages which are deemed sexist, such as the word 'chairman'. But in theology, there are trickier problems. For example, G-d/God is often described in the Bible as 'the God of Abraham, Isaac and Jacob' (see Exodus 3:16), but not 'the God of Sarah, Rebekah and Rachel'. Another example is the book of Proverbs. The book excludes advice to young women, focusing instead only on young men who seek wisdom.

There are examples of similar *androcentrism* in the New Testament as well. For example, in I Corinthians 14:34, St. Paul says that women 'should keep silent' in the church. Women are told to 'be subject to your husbands as to the Lord' (Ephesians 5:22–24). To change the language of patriarchy in Holy Scriptures (Christian or otherwise) may only disguise the misogyny embedded in it. Changing the language will not necessarily remove the patriarchal bias because the patterns and images are arguably part of our subconscious and deep memory.

Recent events in the evangelical community – particularly the release of a gender-inclusive Bible, the TNIV translation (Today's New International Version, 2002) – have raised new concerns over gender and language. For example, does Jesus ask his followers to be fishers of people or fishers of men (Matthew 4:19)? Is there a difference between people and men? Religious women have constantly needed to ask themselves if scriptural references to 'man', 'men' and 'him' actually include them. Other phrases in traditional Christian hymns like 'Good Christian Men Rejoice' or 'Rise Up, O Men of God' are similarly problematic; are these hymns for men or for everyone? Many hymns were written before gender issues entered public consciousness, but their continued use raises concerns. In many cases, we are to assume 'men' is used generically to include everyone – but feminist scholars question that assumption. Surely some aspects of the faith include women while others do not. Some instructions seem to be given to both men and women, but some only to women ('submit to your husbands') and some only to men ('Men, love your wives') (see Jule, 2005).

Other concerns related to *gender-inclusive language* or gender neutral language, focus on the metaphors used for G-d, God or Allah. Some metaphors such as 'rock' and 'fortress' are abstract and poetic; others, such as 'father' and 'son', are anthropomorphic or personal or masculine. Feminist theologians wonder why feminine metaphors have not been emphasized in sermons or Bible studies, since they have also been used throughout the Bible. For example, the Old Testament refers to God as 'a mother bird' (Psalm 17:8b), 'a mother bear' (Hosea 13:8a) and 'a midwife' (Psalm 22:9). There are numerous similar examples of the Holy One being portrayed as feminine throughout traditional scriptures; but, perhaps more important than what gender the Divine is portrayed as is an understanding of the Holy One as both transcendent and removed from human gender boundaries. If the Holy One is limitless, then using human metaphors to explain the nature of G-d, God, Allah will always be problematic. That is to say, God is neither male nor female, but is both; God is transcendent. Metaphorical references to God demonstrate just how deeply language choices matter in forming belief systems.

Gender and Expressions of Morality

In her influential book, *In a Different Voice*, Carol Gilligan (1982) explored gendered language patterns, including gendered patterns of expressing morality. For Gilligan, morality appears closely, if not entirely, connected with one's sense of obligation and one's view of personal sacrifice. She suggests that masculine morality is generally concerned with the public world of social performance and influence, while feminine morality is more often restricted to the private and personal realm. As a result, the moral judgments and moral behaviors and expressions of men tend to differ from those of women.

Gilligan subscribes to the gender-as-difference perspective. In light of Gilligan's ideas, she sees individuals who participate in religious life being encouraged to 'perform' gender. In this context, masculine behavior is connected with public displays of influence while feminine behavior is displayed more intimately, privately and quietly. Religious men are rehearsed into the role of performer and speaker, while women are often rehearsed into and valued in the role of supportive, silent audience members. Women's silence demonstrates to themselves and others a devoutness to the faith, because it is understood to signal their support. Their silence is their way of being good.

One might have thought that the current increased participation of women in Christian theological education, the rise of feminist theology and the growth of women's ordination would have significantly changed the nature of theological education in particular. However, recent research into the lives of evangelical women who chose theological education indicates that the lived experiences of these women are often painful and confusing

(Gallagher, 2003; Ingersoll, 2003; Mutch, 2003). With various other religious experiences possible (including none at all), some women appear to remain and invest in their evangelical subculture because they experience it as something meaningful and worthwhile (Jule, 2006). Women who study theology say they are often dismissed as working against their own purposes, as anti-woman, for pursuing theology at all. Still others feel marginalized, limited and nervous about their possible future contributions to church life; they anticipate problems even if they have not yet experienced any (Mutch, 2003).

Canadian women in theological education report that being a woman in ministry requires 'commitment of conviction' which is carried out within a constant 'context of challenge' (Busse, 1998). Most cite both loneliness and stress as central aspects of their career choice. Nevertheless, women continue to enroll in theological education to graduate and to go on to seek ordination. They choose such struggle. My own research at a theological college revealed how quiet women can be in some Christian settings and how their reasons for this silence are connected to their religious identity (Jule, 2005).

The 1980s and 1990s saw anti-feminism emerge in American society, specifically found inside religious circles (what Susan Faludi, 1993, called 'the backlash'). In spite of early feminist claims made by Christian women in the 1800s and early 1900s, the current American Christian 'right' asserts political pressure on issues concerning the family in direct opposition to feminist causes. It seems that now religious communities articulate a view of society which rejects liberalism and equality in favour of certainty and moral conservatism. Many religious men and women believe they achieve morality and peace of mind by behaving in stereotypically masculine and feminine ways: men to lead, women to submit to male leadership. Though some women may have emotional or intellectual difficulty in such a context, many appear to remain and further invest themselves precisely because of a sense of belonging to a community. They work out their gender roles within a specific framework of male leadership and domination.

The Myth of Gender

What makes gender such an interesting issue in the world religions is the tension of women's fundamental worth: are women inferior to men because God/Jesus/Mohammed were male? Determining an answer is complex. The early Church view of the Virgin Mary emphasized women as docile bodies to be acted upon – that the female body is a site of male power and dominion. Other images and iconography display the Church as 'the bride of Christ', only to be acted upon and claimed by a Christ/male figure. The arguments that see women as different but equal in the church have been used by some theologians to defend women's subordination to men – in general as something natural and God-given. Men are seen as initiators and in the role of 'head', while women are perceived to be nurturers and in the role of 'heart'. Subscribers to this view perceive women who step outside this role to be disobedient, radical and unharmonious. Many women themselves, often those who are part of conservative/traditionalist communities and who express their right and desire to be nurturers in homes that are led by 'strong' men, internalize this view of subordinate women. They see women who seek positions of power as working against their 'authentic womanhood'.

An alternative view, but one which also subscribes to the 'naturally subordinate woman' tradition is 'rooted in the Victorian romanticized myth of females as the morally superior sex' (Walsh, 2001: 170). This view also draws on the Virgin Mary as the ideal woman; her submission brought an enriched spiritual life and purpose. Submission is the higher, better calling. In this view, a public, more powerful role for women demeans them: they are too good for it. Even if women take positions of leadership in the Church, they would make radically different leaders because of their softer, gentler natures. One underlying assumption here is that power is more comfortable – to both men and women – in the hands of men. Women are better equipped to be supporters, not leaders.

Gender Issues in Islam

One of the most visible issues concerning Islam and gender is the wearing of the hijab. Is the wearing of the hijab a choice for women or imposed from within the culture as a requirement for fully enacting a Muslim identity? Muslim women may freely choose to wear the hijab or other coverings for a variety of reasons. Some women wear the hijab because they (or their fathers or husbands) believe that God has instructed women to wear it as a form of modesty. Wearing the hijab is a choice or demand that is made after puberty and is intended to reflect personal devotion to Allah/God. In many cases, the wearing of a headscarf is often accompanied by the wearing of loose-fitting, non-revealing clothing, also referred to as hijab.

While some Muslim women do not perceive the hijab to be obligatory to their faith and don't wear it, other Muslim women wear the hijab as a means of visibly expressing their Muslim or national/cultural identity (Haddad, 2007). In many Islamic nations, the hijab is required whenever the woman is out in public or in the presence of men other than her husband. In many parts of Western society, the hijab is perceived to be synonymous with Islam. By wearing the hijab, some Muslim women hope to communicate their political and social alliance with their country of origin and challenge the prejudice of Western discourses towards the Arabic-speaking world (Zayzafoon, 2005). The wearing of the hijab can also be used to challenge Western feminist discourses which present hijab-wearing women as oppressed or silenced by a male-dominated religion.

The Qur'an views women and men to be equal in human dignity, but, as with Christianity, this equality has not been reflected in the lived practice of the religion. For example, in Islam, women do not have equal rights to make independent decisions about selecting a marriage partner or getting a divorce or maintaining custody of their children. Some Islamic feminists try hard to change Muslim laws to better reflect the full dignity of women, a movement called 'Framework for Progressive Islam'. The biggest frustration for Muslim feminists seems to be the select verses in the Qur'an where certain words and language support patriarchy (like 4:3, which refers to men as 'guardians' of women). Reformists and feminists argue that this concept of guardianship has formed the particularly gendered roles in Muslim societies. In these societies, women are expected to be obedient wives and mothers. They are required to stay within the family environment where men can best protect them. The argument is the issue of guardianship as meaning something more like 'being provided for' than being in the role of a child in need of protection. Feminists see the concept of guardianship as creating rigid divisions of gender roles, with men having social control over women (Hassan, 1996; Wadud, 2005).

A major issue in this debate is sexuality, and the idea that sexuality needs to be controlled. Rigid gender roles and male control over women's sexuality serve as tools to both impose and enforce heterosexuality (Dunn & Kellison, 2010; Mernisse, 2002). Moreover, male heterosexual fantasies seem central to the faith (with references to paradise), with no mention of women's sexuality in a similar way. There are verses which affirm men's rights to sexual satisfaction and allow polygamy and temporary marriage. Women's sexuality in Muslim laws and societies is limited to monogamous heterosexual marriage. This set form of sexuality is believed to be preserving a 'sexual purity' that requires male control over women's sexuality. In some cases where a woman is considered to have violated the codes that keep her or her family's 'sexual purity', her identity or behavior can and has led to so-called honor crimes, resulting in forced marriage, violence or so-called 'honor killings'.

Some scholars believe that these male notions of guardianship and sexuality include the idea that female sexuality, if not controlled, results in social chaos and social disorder. Many reformists and feminist scholars have argued that the Qur'an does not speak specifically to male control of women's sexuality. They have sought to challenge the idea that Islam needs fixed gender roles and contended that the fixation on gender roles impedes women from controlling their own sexuality.

The relationship of any religion and genderedness is politically fascinating. Words and images used for God reflect a particular understanding of the Divine. Those who have a religious faith connect notions of goodness with gender performances so that masculinity is displayed as initiating and central, while femininity is viewed as receptive and required to support men. Does religious faith relate goodness to specific gender performances? Are religious experiences gendered? If there are gendered ways to be moral, are there also gendered ways to be immoral? The specific use of certain words, phrases and textual interpretation of scriptures link to such views. The ways people speak in religious communities connect with genderedness, making religious groups and religious identities a compelling site within which to explore gender alongside language use.

Summing Up

- Religion works alongside gender identity in particular ways, influencing the views of gender inclusion or exclusion and influencing gendered behaviors of belonging.
- Holy Scriptures and traditions seem to both support the oppression and the liberation of women. Interpretations of key passages are sites of debate.
- Though women participate in religious life, religious leadership has been mainly male-dominated; this has influenced the interpretation of scriptures as well as the promotion of androcentric imagery.

7

Gender and Language Use in Relationships

. . . .

There is no female mind. The brain is not an organ of sex.
We may as well speak of a female liver.

Charlotte Perkins Gilman,
Women and Economics

Traditionally, researchers of language and gender have necessarily distingui-
shed between what is known as *institutional talk*, and what is regarded as ordinary, everyday language. In the workplace, in classrooms, or in other public
places, language is often orientated to a goal or task of some sort: this use of
language is institutional talk. But at home and in more personal relationships,
language is used for the establishment and maintenance of relationships. This
chapter explores the role of social talk in personal relationships, and the ways in
which language and gender relate and are used in friendships and in family life.

The Role of Social Talk

Bonnie McElhinny (1998) problematizes this dichotomy of 'ordinary'
versus 'institutional' language. She links public and private contexts and
emphasizes 'the separation rather than the interpenetration of spheres'
(p. 108). McElhinny demonstrates that this distinction between public and
private gets blurry in certain circumstances. Social talk (at home and in
one's personal relationships) is in many ways 'ordinary talk'; yet many workplaces rely on this more casual and friendly style to achieve work-related
goals, and many personal relationships can also function as task-groups.
Deborah Tannen (1990) describes social talk used in places of business
to create rapport among staff for the purposes of conducting effective

business. Also, Shari Kendall (2006) explores how female managers tend to use social talk honed in their personal relationships to create a relaxed work environment. Both Tannen (1990, 1995, 1998) and Janet Holmes (2003, 2006, 2013) have considered how higher-ranking women tell stories at work for the purposes of sustaining authority by framing and positioning their identities as more personal. To some extent, social talk creates rapport and negotiates the status of participants in personal relationships in particular. As such, institutional talk and personal talk are arbitrary distinctions. The context and the people contribute entirely to the *register* of language used.

Eleanor Maccoby (1990) suggested that sex differences only emerged in primarily social situations and not at work. In early childhood, children find same-sex friends more compatible. As children move into adolescence, the patterns they developed in their childhood friendships are carried over into cross-sex encounters, where girls' interactive styles may put them at a disadvantage when it comes to the workplace. Maccoby (1990) found that gender segregation is a widespread phenomenon found in all cultures. Preschool children spend a great deal of their time engaged in activities that are gender-neutral or in same-sex friendships; as they age, their interests diverge along gender lines. Why does this happen? Maccoby suggests that 'peer groups are the setting in which children first discover the compatibility of same-sex others, in which boys first discover the requirements of maintaining one's status in the male hierarchy, and in which the gender of one's partners becomes supremely important' (p. 519).

In mixed-gendered conversations, the variation in speaking style can lead to misunderstandings – at least this was the contention of linguistic scholars in the 1990s. A woman talking to a male friend may interpret his infrequent positive minimal responses as a sign that he is not interested in what she is saying, while to him, he might be trying hard to listen carefully before signaling agreement. To the scholars writing in the 1990s, these misunderstandings emerged from the socialization experienced throughout childhood. On the other hand, a man receiving frequent nods and 'mhms' from his female interlocutor may interpret this as a sign of agreement when, to her, it may merely indicate that she is listening. Daniel Maltz and Ruth Borker (1998) use this example to help explain a common complaint in male–female interaction: men think women agree with them, and women think men aren't agreeing with them. Maltz and Borker conclude that there are 'two separate rules for conversation maintenance which come into conflict and cause massive miscommunication' (p. 422). This view aligns with Difference Theory – that men and women form their own sub-cultures during childhood in same-sex peer groups. Maltz and Borker suggest that these conversation patterns are 'learned in childhood and carried over into adulthood as the bases for patterns of single-sex friendship relations and [...] miscommunication in cross-sex interaction' (p. 423). In their estimation, women's conversation is interactional; men's is more report-based. These views have given way to newer ideas concerning the intersections of gender, social class, race, age, sexual identity, ability, religious background, etc.

Rachel Rafelman (1997) reported in *Toronto Life* magazine how it is that men and women divide along gender lines while both men and women find women more interesting to talk to at parties, because many women have a more developed interactive style. Rafelman refers to women as 'the social grease people' because of their 'training' in drawing people out and getting others to talk about themselves (what Fishman, 1983, referred to as *linguistic shitwork*). Rafelman also suggests that women rarely assert themselves in mixed social settings while enabling others, and so males often dominate these conversations. Rafelman says that, from early childhood, females are spoken to differently than males, and so the content of their speech is distinct with their opinions expressed more obliquely. It seems even highly confident women temper their speech with back-channel support (e.g. 'Oh really', 'How fascinating'). They tend to nod, smile and keep their gaze on the speaker's face. It also seems to be that listening is an important aspect of 'girl talk' since it is at the center of reciprocal communication.

Participating in Family Life

We all create and maintain certain roles for a variety of purposes, and so we have diverse ways of participating in the various relationships in our lives. Kendall (2006) argues that at each moment in any encounter, we take up, resist and assign positions by locating ourselves and others in relation to various values or characteristics, including such social categories as mother, father, sister, son and daughter. There are various discourses and ways of speaking and behaving. There are also different topics and subject positions available in different family groupings. We participate in relationships at home because of the available positions we hold. We may speak in certain ways and about certain things in one role (say, as a daughter) and then quite differently and about different topics altogether in another role (say, as a mother).

Kendall (2006) also points to the role of caregiver as often being that of a woman's. The archetype is based on often non-factual ideals, as Stephanie

Coontz (2003) suggests in her work on American families and the 'myths' that propel them. Our participation in family life reflects the patterns we see in society, and the speech patterns of society are reflected in family life: women tending to children, men tending to financial provision, etc. Even in dual-income homes, many women perform a *second shift*, doing at least twice as much housework and childcare as their partners, because of their traditional role of caretakers in the home (see Bianchi, 2000; Coltrane, 2000). Regardless of career, women still manage the domestic front, and many see their usefulness in line with related domestic tasks.

Family members create and maintain gendered identities, such as the paternal identities of mother and father, through linguistic habits. Kendall (2006) focuses on the 'display through positioning' that family members 'take up'. Her work searches for such displays. For example, she sees that women tend to use individualized topics over generalized topics when at home and in family conversations while men tend to view situations as general. Here's an example:

> Elaine (the mother): Beth just really wants a dog, but uh
> Richard (the father): Oh yeah?
> Elaine: Yeah.
> Richard: Every kid does, I think. Most of them.

(p. 187)

By referring to 'every kid', Richard generalizes the topic to connect with the world beyond family life, while Elaine has individualized the issue to focus on her own daughter. Consequently, Elaine takes the clear parental position, while Richard responded in a way that anyone could have. Such patterns seem to align with gendered roles and expectations; women stay focused on the particulars of their family members, while the masculine habit is to perceive life as beyond the immediacy of family members.

There are other linguistic tendencies which, Kendall (2006) argues, work in similar ways to position the mother as the one most responsible for child-rearing and the father in the role of 'breadwinner' and less emotionally engaged with family matters. Mothers often attempt to frame the conversations as symmetrical exchanges of family experiences, while fathers position themselves as less engaged than mothers. In taking up the position of 'breadwinner', a man constructs a work identity and a greater commitment to life outside the home. Following from these observations, Kendall sees language as creating and reproducing gendered identities that strongly align with work-related identities.

For some theorists, it seems women tend to think in terms of closeness and support, and they are apt to focus on preserving intimacy in their personal relationships. By contrast, men are more likely to focus on independence from family relationships. These traits can lead women and men to starkly different views of the same situation. Deborah Tannen (1990) gave the example of a woman who would check with her husband before inviting a guest to stay because she liked telling friends that she had to check with him (not because she really had to). Her husband, meanwhile, invited people over without consulting his wife because consulting her would mean a loss of his independent status. For social constructivists, such tendencies get rehearsed and performed throughout our lives as we move through various relationships: we behave in certain ways out of a need and desire to be perceived in certain ways by others. We project an image of ourselves that we believe will be positive and acceptable to those we care most about. This approval connects strongly with our genderedness and the gender as we wish to represent: we are approved of in family roles in highly gendered ways. This interpretation of gender and relationships suggests that our performances of genderedness leads to an internalization of these traits: we become what we do and we do what we say.

Gender and Friendships

Friendships allow us the opportunity to partake in relationships based on choice rather than on kinship. By making friends, we assert our autonomy: we choose who to spend time with. The most blatant obstacle to female friendship is the prevailing patriarchal adage that 'women are their own worst enemies'. However, it is by promoting this view that we ensure that women will be each other's worst enemies. Valerie Hey (1996) believed that the friendships of girls, while sometimes affirming, are often times sites of pain and betrayal. Because of internalized misogyny, girls and, later, women work against each other and compete for a whole host of successes, including not only male attention but also other female friendships, and appearance. Janice Raymond (1985) saw that, instead of engagement with more worldly concerns, women engage in an over-concern for their own lives. Raymond's research points to ways some women use talk at the center of their relationships as a form of therapy where women come to believe that what really counts in their life is the search for health and happiness and their ability to articulate this. In this way, women use their friendships as therapy. A key way this therapeutic relationship is developed is through mutual self-disclosure. Female friendships require girls and women to 'show and tell' everything. Raymond calls this a 'psychological strip-tease' that can fragment and exploit the inner life. The relationship-centeredness of many women makes other people the center of a woman's life rather than the self. When a relationship ends, all else fails.

There has also been increased scholarly interest in boys' friendships and the role these play in establishing acceptable masculine identities. 'Boy culture' seems to be established through actions and shared activity (Pollack, 1998). According to this view, boys are particularly motivated to avoid shame and to increase athletic ability. Research has also explored what boys and men talk about in their friendship groups (Cameron, 2005; Coates, 1996), suggesting that boys are very similar to each other, often discussing similar topics in their friendship groups and sharing openly. This possibility interrupts the earlier claims of essential difference between female and male in this regard.

Jennifer Coates (1996) has done a considerable amount of research on linguistic patterns in female friendship groups, or what she calls social networks. She identifies a range of linguistic features in social networks, such as: topic and topic introduction; latching; minimal response; hedging; questions; and turn-taking. These features are underpinned by Coates' belief that female speech (if it exists) is not weak at all, but, rather, is a style of speaking that is based on a goal of 'maintenance of good social relationships' (p. 139).

Coates believes that different conversational settings might require varying levels of competition over relationship-building speech patterns for both males and females. Female conversations may more often be relationship/community based even though 'the ideal (androgynous) speaker would be competent in both [settings]' (p. 139). Deborah Jones (1980) categorized female friendship discourse into four main themes:

- House talk: the exchange of information and resources connected with the female role as an occupation.
- Scandal: the talk about the behavior of others, and of women in particular. It is usually made in terms of the domestic morality of which women have been appointed guardians.
- Bitching: the overt expression of women's anger at their restricted roles or inferior status. They express this frustration in private and to other women only. The women who 'bitch' are not expecting change; they want only to make their complaints in an environment where their anger will be understood and expected.

- Chatting: the most intimate form of gossip, a mutual self-disclosure, a transaction where women use to their own advantage the skills they have learned as a part of their job of nurturing others.

Such themes frame conversations in many female friendships so that they become feminine 'scripts'. Jones suggested that failure to engage with these themes excluded a woman from full connectedness with her female friends. With her friendship network, a woman would utilize the themes of House talk, Scandal, Bitching and Chatting to connect, affirm and protect the friendship. This social talk seems to be the connective tissue for most women in their friendship groups.

One in-depth look at female friendships is Kate Fillion's (1996) book, *Lip Service*. Fillion provided insights into how close girlfriends relate to one another and why men are so criticized for not making friends in a similar way. The gist of it is that intimacy has been defined in a feminine way so that women come out as the *de facto* intimacy experts over men. Such ideas echo the earlier ideas of Tannen's (1990) and Gilligan's (1982) that stated that self-disclosure is the defining feature of female intimacy – that women measure closeness by how much personal disclosure transpires. Julia Wood (1997) connected this idea to how men are judged to be less adept at intimacy because they fail to emphasize the personally disclosive talk that characterizes women's relationships.

In Wood's (1997) research, more men said that they demonstrate affection by doing things for and with others, but this activity-based frame was not similar to the definitions of intimacy for women. Women said they demonstrated affection by telling others about their feelings, and they received higher approval from women as a direct result. Men told researchers that they feel close to their friends through 'mutual give and take', 'helping each other out', 'being there' and 'sharing activities'. Women said that these demonstrations did not matter as much to them in their friendships as self-disclosure.

Deborah Cameron (1995) says that wherever and whenever the matter of masculine/feminine relations has been investigated, both women and men have been found to face normative expectations about the appropriate mode of speech for their assumed gender. Both men and women have been instructed and rehearsed (by themselves and each other) in the most acceptable ways of talking, just as they have been instructed in the most acceptable ways of dressing or behaving to align with a *normative* genderedness. Cameron labels their acceptance of a 'proper' speech style *verbal hygiene*.

She claims that verbal hygiene is a way society makes sense of language and a symbolic attempt to impose order on the social world. We belong when we play by the relevant gender rules.

Politeness and Complimenting

Of relevance to the topic of politeness is the work of Janet Holmes (1995, 2003) and her theory of politeness in the workplace language. Her data suggest that all people tend to be more polite both to people who are socially superior (or strategically important to them) and to strangers. Holmes connects women's experiences at the workplace as often in positions of support rather than leadership – that they are in relationships at work as working for those who are socially superior (like with their bosses) or with strangers. Quite simply, women get more practice with polite talk on a daily basis because in their many roles, they are often in an inferior position, or they are in familial or relational roles.

Janet Holmes (2003) has also done much work on complimenting, identifying three types of compliments: compliments related to appearance ('What a lovely dress'); compliments in the form of greetings ('How good to see you here'); and expressions of concern ('You seem to be much stronger'). Holmes maintains that giving praise in these ways is inherently asymmetrical; the speaker is attempting to 'one-up' the other. Her data from TV talk shows indicates that women give 70% of compliments and receive about 75% of them. Compliments between men are rare – less than 10%. This discrepancy suggests that women are giving compliments to each other and, as a result, are recipients of all manner of social judgments. According to Holmes, the way a woman is spoken to is a subtle and powerful means of perpetuating her subordinate role in society. Like giving praise to a child, such complimenting can be patronizing.

Holmes's research specifically explores how women are complimented on their appearance and behavior while men are more likely to be complimented on their abilities and possessions. She provides evidence of men being more likely to pay compliments to women only if the woman is on par or of higher status. As such, Holmes sees women as complimented most by their equals and their peers and friends, as a way of connecting with each other and perhaps also to control each other for the purposes of self-affirmation.

Additionally, female friendships in particular are complex sites where a feminine style of speaking (such as using back-channel support, latching or listening) can 'ghettoize' women, inadvertently limiting a wider set of experiences. Women connect with each other through conversation but, within these conversations, women also use language to narrow the focus onto personal lives rather than outside local or more global issues. Their friendships serve as sites of support, but also as sites of exclusion.

Rosalind Wiseman (2002) explored the pain at the center of many female friendships in adolescence in her book, *Queen Bees and Wannabees*. Here she explores the dynamics of peer groups and the power games that play out within them. Rachel Simmons (2002) also examines female friendships in her book, *Odd Girl Out*, and identifies the 'hidden aggression' inside female friendship groups. Because of such explorations, we can no longer view women as simply the nurturers: gender roles are too complex for simple generalizations. In addition, experiences shift from one generation to another, and from one circumstance to another.

Talk used in personal relationships reveals a social construction of gender as well as alignments of gendered patterns, in keeping with a Difference perspective. Because the role of men in Western society has been and continues to be work-based, these patterns are carried into personal relations at home and in friendship groups. That said, personal relationships are centered around feelings of belonging and participation regardless of one's sex. How people behave in their personal relations seems to closely align with gender differentiated ways of communicating with the world at large: women tend to build rapport with others through conversations, and men tend to function as individuals more disengaged from personal relationships.

Summing Up

- The gendered roles we play in our personal relationships are often revealed in linguistic practices; for example, women tend to individualize topics while men tend to generalize and distance themselves from the context.
- Both women and men have been instructed and rehearsed into the acceptable ways of talking in order to align with a particular gender identity. We behave in certain ways because we are comfortable doing so.
- The role of language in various relationships, including at home, in friendship groups and in workplaces, serves two purposes: to affirm and to control others.

8

An Anti-Conclusion

. . . .

Feminism is as relevant as it ever was. In the last few years
we have been excited by a vibrant feminist movement which seems
to be growing exponentially.

Redfern and Aune

I've called this concluding chapter an anti-conclusion because of the reality that the issues and situations discussed in this book will never end. There can never be a conclusion to this critical area of inquiry. Because time and place are so transient, no reasonable conclusions are ever possible.

Very broadly speaking, this book has focused on two things:

1. How language reveals, represents, constructs and sustains attitudes to gender, and
2. How language users speak in ways that contribute to their gendered-inflected lives.

Both of these topics include historical influences, past views of what makes a good woman or man, and a recognition that language is used to control or connect everyone in some way. Studying language can and must be objective insofar as we can assess, record and reflect on language, even though studying gender can be so subjective and personally experienced.

The issues of nature or nurture, or heredity/biology and environment, connect with the media, education, workplace, religious communities, family patterns and social conditioning. Each individual is a mysterious and unique combination of compounding social factors. However, there seem to be some persistent language patterns that align with gender. Studying gender and language is interesting in large part because we often want to find support for our developing views or life experiences. It can be very easy to use the claims made by linguists in the past to explain our present circumstances, but such ventures can also be unsatisfactory because research done in specific communities from the 1960s to the 1990s may not relate to our current circumstances. Though much more research has emerged in the last 20 years or so, foundational feminist work in this area of inquiry does seem to emerge earlier.

It is certainly important to caution all of us against adopting entrenched positions or easily or quickly dismissing ideas on the basis of personal experiences only. Any attempt to divide the world into two sexes with no common ground should certainly be resisted. The world is complex and we, as participants in it, are not easily categorized or predictable. It seems to me after a lifetime of reflection on the matter that more and more evidence always serves to make the relationship of gender and language use more complex. This intricacy must be continually explored because it is in constant flux. In this way, researchers are consistently searching out new sites and new research results in the quest to understand language and gender.

In looking at language, it is helpful for us to consider that the consensus view of gender makes an impact on the way we live out our lives. However, this impact is not universal because people make choices in various settings and for a variety of reasons to perform in certain gendered ways – or to reject those performances. I believe that we all have been rehearsed into various gender performances for a range of reasons, and that the rehearsal is closely connected to language. We grow up inside families, religious or non-religious communities, schools, and particular cultures, ethnicities, positions and worldviews. We cannot fully define ourselves – others play significant roles in determining who we are.

The centrality of gender to how we live our lives, what choices we make, who we befriend and connect with is part of understanding the connection. Would I still be myself if I were born male? How central is my sex to my gender identity? Would I still be myself if I were born elsewhere? I think that my life trajectory would be different because of the myriad ways society would treat me and reward certain behaviors and attitudes. My being born female influenced my early experiences with others. Since I am a cisgendered person I am viewed as feminine by the world around me. And this set of circumstances and the heteronormative world that surrounds me frame many of my life experiences.

The rise of feminism has opened up the lives of women around the world to include connection to experiences beyond family life. But this journey has not been quick or painless. Many thinkers, philosophers, politicians and researchers have explored the boundaries of gender roles and gender tendencies in speech that continue to surround both sexes and create such distinct life experiences in the workplace and in personal relationships. We are all here, on planet earth, all sharing its joys and responsibilities alongside each other. We need the full range of gender identities to humanize our lived experiences. We are each capable of strength and responsiveness, independence and interdependence, competitiveness and collaboration, masculine and feminine.

It is my opinion, at least at the moment, that 'differences' are not the problem in our lives. We live with who we are. What are problems, and problems worth engaging with, are gender polarization, gender binaries and the tension between perceived differences. Perhaps we need to use other words other than 'difference' (which creates and supports a narrow gender binary) – words like 'tapestry' of gender or 'symphony' of gender so as to better conceptualize gender identity as a mixture of various styles and purposes. I wonder if the next 10 years will see a shift in these concepts.

As stated at the beginning of this book, I am fascinated by how much of an effect gender and language use have had on my own life choices, my self-concept and identity, and my relationships with others. I can appreciate that socialization is powerful and insidious; but I also appreciate that we are also powerful, exist with complex combinations of past and present situations, and possess our own agency in a host of various circumstances.

I also wonder what kind of world we want: a divided, 'ghettoized' society where masculinity and femininity are divisions, or one where people are recognized to be wholly worthwhile, regardless of their age, life stage, faith, color, class, gender identity or sex? Language use in the media, education, the workplace, our faith communities, and our personal relationships matter a great deal in creating and then protecting a world we want. Thoughtfulness surrounding these spaces and our roles within them is what is needed.

There are many areas of enquiry I have not explored here, namely gender and language use in politics, the law, in sports, in psychological development, in aging, or in various cultures around the world of course, there is much research in these areas, but there is much potential for more research. There is also so much more to say on the topics discussed in this book and so much more complexity to discuss. I hope you find your own way to explore a plethora of possibilities and ideas. Perhaps, at the very least, this book has given you some new ways of looking at the circumstances surrounding you. The field is open wide to those who come with new questions and insights – so feel free to join in. I hope the topics introduced here have given you a sense of the field of gender and language use, along with some key notions and concepts within it that you will continue to ponder throughout your life.

Finally, I want to say that I continue to contemplate how gender influences our lived experiences. Women are still the usual victims of domestic violence abuse and sexual harassment at schools and in the workplace; women are more often than not the victims of the media's use of ideal images; older women are more disregarded than older men; women are still socialized to be dependent and enmeshed, while men are socialized to seek autonomy and power over others. Around the world, women are more often victims of rape, prostitution and infanticide. In some places, women are the property of men, and poverty is largely a women's issue. I am troubled by the ways our gender marks us and limits our possibilities. My ultimate hope is that an increased awareness of gender and language use will open up our own understandings of human connection, and that our experiences will be fuller because of it.

Glossary

. . . .

Agency One's capacity to originate and direct one's own actions in response to the individual's surrounding environment or contexts.

Androcentric Describing the practice, conscious or otherwise, of placing male human beings or the masculine point of view at the center of one's view of the world.

Baby-boomers Those born during any period of increased birth rate, but particularly applied to those born during the post-World War II period and before the Vietnam War. In Europe, it is also known as the Generation of 1968.

Biological determinism The hypothesis that biological factors such as one's individual genes (as opposed to social or environmental factors) completely determine how one behaves or changes over time. It is the opposite of social determinism.

Cisgendered A term for someone who has a gender identity that aligns with the sex they were assigned at birth (i.e. non-transgendered people).

Complementarian A term used to describe a theological view that an unequal position of men and women, particularly in marriage and in church leadership, is biblically required. The term replaces what previously was known as the Traditionalist view of gender relationships.

Consciousness raising groups A form of political action pioneered by radical feminists in the United States in the late 1960s. The groups of women aimed to achieve a better understanding of women's oppression, among a wider group of citizens, by bringing women together to discuss and analyze their lives without interference from the presence of men.

Consumer femininity – see Consumer gender.

Consumer gender The study of how people buy, what they buy, when they buy, and why they buy in alignment with gender stereotypes and gender identity. Researchers in this area attempt to understand the buyer decision-making process in gender groupings.

Consumer masculinity – see Consumer gender.

Creaky voice A special kind of phonation in which the arytenoid cartilages in the larynx are drawn together.

Critical Discourse Analysis (CDA) An interdisciplinary approach to the study of discourse which views language as a form of social practice; it focuses on the ways social and political domination/power is reproduced by text and talk. The patterns of access to communicative events is an essential element of CDA.

Cultivation theory The effect TV and film have on society and how consumption cultivates a distorted perception of real life.

Egalitarian The moral doctrine that people should be treated as equals. Generally, it applies to the notion that all individuals should be held equal under the law and the Church, and is particularly concerned with gender roles and contributions.

Equal Rights Amendment A proposed amendment to the United States Constitution that was intended to guarantee equal rights under the law for Americans regardless of sex, but it failed to pass Congress approval in 1979 and again in 1982.

Essentialism The view that, for any specific kind of entity, it is at least theoretically possible for there to be a set of characteristics shared by all members of a specified group.

Feminine/Femininity Refers to qualities and behaviors judged by a particular culture to be ideally associated with or especially appropriate to women and girls. In Western culture, femininity has traditionally included features such as gentleness and patience.

Gender Refers to the social construction of behaviors in alignment with 'masculine' or 'feminine', rather than the biological condition of maleness or femaleness. The term is often used interchangeably with sex, but in the social sciences 'gender' refers to socioculturally adapted traits.

Gender bias – see Sexism.

Gender-inclusive language (or gender-neutral or politically-correct language) A description of language usages aimed at minimizing assumptions regarding the biological sex of human referents and directed at clarifying the inclusion of both sexes and genders.

Gender roles A set of perceived behavioral norms associated particularly with males or females in a given social group or system, and often a focus for analysis in the social sciences. All societies have a gender/sex system, although the components and workings of these systems vary widely from society to society.

Gendered Feminine or masculine ways of behaving.

The glass ceiling Refers to situations where the advancement of a person within the hierarchy of an organization is limited. 'Glass' refers to the limitation as not immediately apparent but rather an unwritten or unofficial policy.

Hegemony Leadership or dominance, especially by one social group over others.

Heteronormative Denoting or relating to a worldview that promotes heterosexuality as the normal or preferred sexual orientation.

Hierarchy A system of ranking and organizing things or people, where each element of the system (except for the top element) is subordinate to a single other element. In gender studies, the hierarchy is usually understood as being male dominated and female subordinated.

Ideal A principle or value that one actively pursues as a goal. In gender studies, the ideal is the gendered values supported by any given society or group.

Institutional talk A type of communication situation taking place between an official and a client of an office in an institutional setting when the asymmetry of the relation is maintained in terms of power.

Intersex A variety of conditions in which a person is born with a reproductive or sexual anatomy that doesn't fit the typical definitions of female or male.

Liberal feminism A form of feminism that argues that equality for women can be achieved through legal means and social reform. Liberal feminism leans towards an equality of sameness with men.

Linguistic shitwork The trivial, unrewarding and tedious parts of conversations that keep the conversation going, like the asking of questions to spark a meaningful discussion.

Linguistic space Refers to the amount of talking taken up by a speaker or speakers in any given conversation. One can take up a lot of linguistic space by saying a lot, while another may take up very little linguistic space by not saying much out loud.

Masculine/Masculinity Refers to qualities and behaviors judged by a particular culture to be ideally associated with or especially appropriate to men. In Western culture, masculinity has traditionally included features such as strength and independence.

Mediated Having brought about a result.

Minorities Groups that do not constitute a politically dominant set of the total population of a given society. A sociological minority is not necessarily a numerical minority; it may include any group that is disadvantaged with respect to a dominant group in terms of social status, education, employment, wealth and/or political power.

Misogyny Hatred or strong prejudice against women as a group and femininity in general. It is often a political ideology that justifies and maintains the subordination of women to men.

National Organization of Women (NOW) An American feminist group founded in 1966 with currently over 500,000 contributing members. During the 1970s in particular, NOW promoted the Equal Rights Amendment to the United States Constitution.

Neoliberalism A modern politico-economic theory favoring free-trade, privatization, minimal government intervention in business, reduced public expenditure on social services, etc.

Non-cisgendered A term used to describe individuals whose sex and gender are not aligned.

Normative/The Norm The term used to describe the effects of those cultural structures which regulate the function of social activity. Also describes actions intended to normalize something or to make something acceptable.

Othering/The Other A key concept that refers to that which is other than oneself. The concept of otherness is integral to the understanding of identities, as people construct roles for themselves in relation to, or as vastly different from, an 'other'.

Patriarchy The ideological structuring of society on the basis of family units in which fathers have primary responsibilities for the welfare of their families and, by extension, the responsibility for the community as a whole. *Note:* opposing the patriarchy has nothing to do with not liking men; it's the societal structures that are of concern here.

Power More or less the unilateral ability (either real or perceived) or potential to bring about significant change through the actions of oneself or of others. The term 'power' is contested by scholars because of the assumptions surrounding who or what has it.

Racism Bigotry, prejudice, violence, oppression, stereotyping, discrimination or any other socially divisive practice whose primary basis is the concept of race. It is also the belief or ideology that all members of each race possess characteristics of abilities specific to that race, especially to distinguish it as being either superior or inferior to another.

Radical feminism A branch of feminism that views women's oppression as a basic system of power upon which human relationships in society are arranged. It seeks to challenge power relations by rejecting standard/traditional gender roles. Radical feminists locate the root cause of women's oppression in patriarchal gender relations, as opposed to legal systems (liberal feminism) or class conflict (socialist feminism).

Register A formality/informality scale concerning the use of language as determined by the situation. (High register is more formal.)

Sapir–Whorf hypothesis An axiom underlying the work of Edward Sapir and Benjamin Whorf in the 1920s which states that there is a systematic relationship between the language a person speaks and how that person both understands the world and behaves in it. The nature of a particular language influences the habitual thought of its speakers.

Second shift In two-career heterosexual couples, men and women on average spend about equal amounts of time working, but women still spend more time on housework (known as her 'second shift'). Several studies provide statistical evidence that married men contribute a smaller share of housework, regardless of whether or not they earn more than their wives.

Secularization To make secular; separate from religious or spiritual connection or influences; to make worldly or unspiritual.

Semiotics The study of meaning-making of signs and symbols as elements of communicative behavior; a general theory of signs and symbolism usually divided into the branches of pragmatics, semantics and syntactics.

Sex Referring to the male and female duality of biology and reproduction. Also a contested term.

Sex differences A distinction of biological and/or physiological characteristics typically associated with either males or females of a species. For example, on average men are taller than women (a sex difference), but an individual woman may be taller than an individual man.

Sex-preferential speech Men and women use distinctive lexical items as well as choose different topics for conversation during an interaction.

Sexism The discrimination and/or hatred against people based on their sex rather than on any individual traits. Can also refer to any and all systemic differentiations based on the sex of the individuals which views either male or female as more superior than the other.

Sexual revolution The liberalization of established social and moral attitudes toward sex, particularly that occurred in Western countries during the 1960s.

Slut-shaming The act of criticizing a woman for her real or presumed sexual activity, or for behaving in ways that someone thinks are associated with her real or presumed sexual activity.

Social construction/Socially constructed Any institutionalized entity or artifact in a social system where its meaning is constructed by participation in a particular culture or society, which itself exists because people agree to behave according to conventional rules.

Social sciences A group of academic disciplines that studies human aspects of the world. Usually includes: anthropology, economics, education, geography, law, linguistics, politics, philosophy, psychology and sociology. These disciplines tend to emphasize the use of the scientific method in the study of humanity, including the use of quantitative and qualitative methods.

Socialist feminism A branch of feminism that focuses upon both the public and private sphere of a woman's life and argues that liberation can only be achieved by working to end both the economic and cultural sources of women's oppression.

Stereotype A widely held but fixed and oversimplified image or idea of a particular type of person or groups of people.

Subject positions A location for people within relationships. A person (a subject) inevitably sees the world from the vantage point of that position.

Subjectivity Refers to the property of perceptions, arguments and language as being based in a subject's point of view, and hence influenced in accordance with a particular bias and related to power relations.

Synthetic sisterhood/Synthetic personalization The process by which texts treat their mass audience as if they were individuals. Magazines, newspapers or other media use linguistic devices such as personal pronouns and presuppositions to construct a simulated friendship between audience member and the producer.

Theory of Deficit or Dominance/Dominance Theory The theory which states that societies are stratified by sex, and that human social hierarchies consist of a hegemonic group at the top, usually men; and that women are dominated by the power of those born male.

Theory of Difference/Difference Theory The theory postulating that there are innate or somewhat socialized differences in the use of language between males and females.

Verbal hygiene A phrase coined by British linguist Deborah Cameron to describe 'the urge to meddle in matters of language': that is, the effort to improve or correct speech and writing.

Vocal fry The vocal fry register (creaky, croaky, popcorning, glottal rattle) is considered a low vocal register and is produced through a loose glottal closure which permits air to bubble through slowly with a rattling sound of a low frequency (also see Creaky voice).

Voice Refers to the authenticity and distinctiveness of someone's spoken or written expression and aligns with the right, the opportunity or the ability to express a choice or opinion.

References

....

Adichie, C.N. (2015) *We Should All Be Feminists*. London: Fourth Estate.

Anderson, D. (2016) *Alberta MLA Sandra Jansen latest long string of female politicians to face abuse*. CBC News on-line. www.cbc.ca/news/Canada/Calgary/sandra-jansen-alberta-mla-misogyny-1.3865047.

Andres, L. (2004) *Student Affairs: Experiencing Higher Education*. Vancouver: UBC Press.

Ardener, S. (2005) Ardener's 'muted groups': The genesis of an idea and its praxis. *Women and Language* 28.2 (Fall 2005) 50–54, 72.

Arquette, R. (2002) *Searching for Debra Winger*. USA: Immortal Entertainment (motion picture).

Badinter, E. (2006) *Dead end Feminism*. Cambridge: Polity Press.

Bakan, A. and Stasiulis, D. (1997) *Not One of the Family: Domestic Workers in Canada*. Toronto: University of Toronto Press.

Baxter, J. (2003) *Positioning Gender in Discourse: A Feminist Methodology*. Basingstoke: Palgrave Macmillan.

Baxter, J. (ed.) (2006) *Speaking Out: The Female Voice in Public Contexts*. Basingstoke: Palgrave Macmillan.

Bechdel, A. (1986) *Dykes to Watch Out For*. Ann Arbor, Michigan: Firebrand Books.

Berekashvili, N. (2012) The role of gender-biased perceptions in teacher-student interaction. *Psychology of Language and Communication* 16 (1), 39–51.

Bianchi, S. (2000) Maternal employment and time with children: Dramatic change or surprising continuity? *Demography* Nov 37 (4), 401–414.

Bindel, J. *Viewpoint: Should gay men and lesbians be bracketed together?* BBC News Magazine. 2 July 2014, www.bbc.com/news/magazine-28130472.

Bing, J.M. and Bergvall, V. (1996) The question of questions: Beyond binary thinking. In V. Bergvall, J.M. Bing and A. Freed (eds) *Rethinking Language and Gender Research*. London: Longman.

Bodine, A. (1975) Androcentrism in prescriptive grammar: Singular 'they,' sex-indefinite 'he,' and 'he or she.' *Language in Society* 4, 129–146.

Bowles, S. and Gintis, H. (2013) *A Cooperative Species: Human Reciprocity and its Evolution*. Princeton, NJ: Princeton University Press.

Brownhill, S., Warin, J. and Wernersson, I. (2015) *Men, Masculinities and Teaching in Early Childhood Education: International Perspectives.* Abingdon, OXON: Routledge.

Bucholtz, M. (2011) *White Kids: Language, Race, and Styles of Youth Identity.* Cambridge: Cambridge University Press.

Bucholtz, M. and Hall, K. (2004) Theorizing identity in language and sexuality research. *Language in Society* 33, 469–515.

Burgess, M., Stermer, S. and Burgess, S. (2007) Sex, lies and video games: The portrayal of male and female characters on video game covers. *Sex Roles* 57 (5/6), 419–433.

Butler, J. (1990) *Gender Trouble: Feminism and the Subversion of Identity.* New York: Routledge.

Bystydzienski, J. and Bird, S.R. (eds) (2006) *Removing Barriers: Women in Academic Science, Technology, Engineering and Mathematics.* Bloomington: Indiana University Press.

Caldas-Coulthard, C. (1996) Women who pay for sex. And enjoy it: Transgression versus morality in women's magazines. In C. Caldas-Coulthard and M. Coulthard (eds) *Texts and Practices: Readings in Critical Discourse Analysis.* London: Routledge.

Cameron, D. (1992) *Researching Language: Issues of Power and Method.* Abingdon, UK: Taylor and Francis.

Cameron, D. (ed.) (1998) *The Feminist Critique of Language* (2nd edn). London: Routledge.

Cameron, D. (2001) *Working with Spoken Discourse.* London: Sage.

Cameron, D. (2005) Language, gender and sexuality: Current issues and new directions. *Applied Linguistics* 26 (4), 482–502.

Cameron, D. (2008) *The Myth of Mars and Venus: Do Men and Women Really Speak Different Languages?* Oxford: Oxford University Press.

Carson, D.A. (1998) *The Inclusive-Language Debate: A Plea for Realism.* Grand Rapids: Baker Books.

Carter, C., Steiner, L. and McLaughlin, L. (eds) (2014) *Routledge Companion to Media and Gender.* New York and London: Routledge.

Charles, C. (2007) Digital media and 'girling' at an elite girls' school. *Learning Media and Technology* 32 (2), 135–147.

Cheshire, J. (2000) The telling or the tale? Narratives and gender in adolescent friendship networks. *Journal of Sociolinguistics* 4, 236–262.

Chopp, R. (1989) *The Power to Speak: Feminism, Language and God.* New York: Crossroad.

Clark, C. (2016) Christy Clark reveals personal reason for supporting sexual assault bill. *Vancouver Sun* 10 June.

Clowes, L., Shefer, T., Fouten, E., Vergnani, T., Jacobs, J. (2009) Coercive sexual practices and gender-based violence on a university campus. *Agenda: Empowering Women for Gender Equity* 23 (80), 22–32.

Coates, J. (1993) *Women, Men and Language* (2nd edn). New York: Longman.

Coates, J. (1996) *Women Talk: Conversation between Women Friends*. Oxford: Blackwell.

Coates, J. (2003) *Men Talk*. Oxford: Blackwell.

Coltrane, S. (2000) Research on household labour: Modeling and measuring the social embeddedness of routine family work. *Journal of Marriage and the Family* November 62 (4), 1208–1233.

Connell, R. (1995) *Masculinities*. Cambridge: Polity.

Coontz, S. (2003) *The Way We Never Were: American Families and the Nostalgia Trap*. New York: Basic Books.

Criado-Perez, C. (2013) Have the police failed to record the Twitter threats against me? *New Statesmen* (blog) 5 September.

Dalhousie University (2014) Gender-neutral washrooms. See http://www.dal.ca (accessed 2 May 2016).

Daly, M. (1973) *The Church and the Second Sex*. New York: Harper and Row.

Davies, J. (2003) Expressions of gender: An analysis of pupils' gendered discourse styles in small group classroom discussions. *Discourse and Society* 14.2 (March), 115–132.

De Beauvoir, S. (1952) *The Second Sex*. New York: Vintage Books.

De Francisco, V. (1991) The sounds of silence: How men silence women in marital relations. *Discourse and Society* 2 (4), 413–423.

Delamont, S. (2012) *Sex Roles and the School* (2nd edn). Abingdon: Routledge.

Dimulescu, C. (2015) *A Theoretical and Practical Approach to Gendered Talk-in-Interaction*. Germany: Scholars' Press/Omniscriptum.

Diprete, T.A. (2013) *The Rise of Women: The Growing Gender Gap in Education and What It Means for American Schools*. New York, NY: Russell Sage Foundation.

Driscoll, B. (2013) Caroline Criado-Perez says Twitter rape threat campaign 'Isn't a feminist issue'. *The Huffington Post* 29 July.

Dunn, S. and Kellison, R.B. At the intersection of scripture and law: Qur'an 4:34 and violence against women. *Journal of Feminist Studies in Religion* 26 (2), 11–36. Indiana University Press. Retrieved June 9, 2016, from Project MUSE database.

Dworkin, A. (1981) *Pornography: Men Possessing Women*. Toronto: Women's Press.

Eastin, M. (2006) Video game violence and the female game player: Self- and opponent gender effects on presence and aggressive thoughts. *Human Communication Research* 32 (2), 351–372.

Eckert, P. and McConnell-Ginet, S. (2013) *Language and Gender* (2nd edn). Cambridge: Cambridge University Press.

Ehrlich, S. (2001) *Representing Rape: Language and Sexual Consent*. New York: Routledge.

Ehrlich, S. and Meyerhoff, M. (2014) Introduction. In S. Ehrlich, M. Meyerhoff and J. Holmes (eds) *The Handbook of Language, Gender and Sexuality* (2nd edn). Oxford: Wiley Blackwell.

Eilperin, J. (2016) White House women want to be in the room where it happens. *The Washington Post* online 13 September.

Elgot, J. (2016) Andrea Leadsom apologizes to Theresa May for motherhood remarks. *The Guardian* 11 July.

Epstein, D., Elwood, J., Hey, V. and Maw, J. (eds) (1998) *Failing Boys? Issues in Gender and Achievement*. Buckingham: Open University Press.

Fairclough, N. (1992) *Discourse and Social Change*. Cambridge: Polity Press.

Fairclough, N. (1995) *Media Discourse*. London: Arnold.

Faludi, S. (1993) *Backlash: The Undeclared War against Women*. New York: Vintage.

Fichtelius, A., Johansson, I. and Nordin, K. (1980) Three investigations of sex-associated speech variation in day school. *Women's International Studies* 3 (2–3), 219–225.

Fillion, K. (1996) *Lip Service: The Myth of Female Virtue in Love, Sex and Friendship*. New York: Harper Collins.

Fisher, B., Cullen, F. and Turner, M. (2000) *The Sexual Victimization of College Women*. Washington, DC: US Department of Justice, Research Report.

Fishman, P. (1983) Interaction: The work women do. In B. Thorne, C. Kramarae, and N. Henley (eds) *Language, Gender and Society*. Rowley, MA: Newbury House.

Flanders, N. (1970) *Analyzing Teacher Behaviour*. Reading, MA: Addison-Wesley.

Foucault, M. (1972) *The Archaeology of Knowledge and Discourse on Language*. New York: Pantheon Books.

Foucault, M. (1978) *The History of Sexuality: An Introduction*. Harmondsworth: Penguin.

Francis, B. (2000) The gendered subject: Students' preferences and discussions of gender and subject ability. *Oxford Review of Education* 26, 35–48.

Furlong, M. (1991) *A Dangerous Delight: Women and Power in the Church.* London: SPCK.

Gallagher, S.K. (2003) *Evangelical Identity and Gendered Family Life.* London, UK: Rutgers University Press.

Gamble, S. (2001) Postfeminism. In *Routledge Companion to Feminism.* New York: Routledge.

Gauntlett, D. (2002) *Media, Gender and Identity: An Introduction.* New York: Routledge.

Gill, R. (2007) *Gender and the Media.* Cambridge, UK: Polity Press.

Gilligan, C. (1982) *In a Different Voice: Psychological Theory and Women's Development.* Cambridge, MA: Harvard University Press.

Girls Who Code: www.girlswhocode.org.

Graddol, D. and Swann, J. (1989) *Gender Voices.* London: Blackwell.

Griffith, R.M. (1997) *God's Daughters: Evangelical Women and the Power of Submission.* Berkeley: University of California.

Gurian, M. and Stevens, K. (2005) *The Minds of Boys: Saving our Sons from Falling Behind in School and Life.* San Francisco: Jossey-Bass.

Haddad, Y.Y. (2007) The post-9/11 hijab as icon. *Sociology of Religion* 68 (3), 253–267.

Hale, S. (2005) *The Goose Girl.* New York: Bayern Books.

Hall, K. and Bucholtz, M. (eds) (1995) *Gender Articulated Language and the Socially Constructed Self.* Oxford: Oxford University Press.

Harris, K.M. (2013) Sexuality and suicidality: Matched pairs analyses reveal unique characteristics in non-heterosexual suicidal behaviours. *Archives of Sexual Behaviour* 42 (5), 729–737.

Hartley, B.L. and Sutton, R.M. (2013) A stereotype threat account of boys' academic achievement. *Child Development* 84 (5), 1716–1733.

Haskins, S. (2013) *Target Women.* 26 January 2016, www.youtube.com.

Hassan, R. (1996) Religious Human Rights in the Qur'an. See. http://www.oozebap.org%2Fbiblio%2FReligious_Human_Rights_in_the_Quran.rtf&usg=AFQjCNEYIwYoMIjzt8EzGRx0gOhHK0wN2g&sig2=R7Y7RC7e5IFAzFub7lSk_g (accessed April 3, 2004).

Helgesen, S. (1995) *The Female Advantage.* New York: Doubleday.

Henderson, E.F. (2015) *Gender Pedagogy: Teaching, Learning and Tracing Gender in Higher Education.* Basingstoke: Palgrave Pivot.

Herrett-Skjellum, J. and Allen, M. (1996) Television programming and sex-stereotyping: A meta-analysis. *Communication Yearbook* 19, 157–185.

Hey, V. (1996) *The Company She Keeps: An Ethnography of Girls' Friendship.* Buckingham: Open University Press.

Holmes, J. (1995) *Women, Men and Politeness.* London: Longman.

Holmes, J. (1998) Women's talk: The question of sociolinguistic universals. In J. Coates (ed.) *Language and Gender: A Reader* (pp. 471–483). Oxford: Blackwell.

Holmes, J. (2000) Politeness, power and provocation: Humour functions in the workplace. *Discourse Studies* 2 (2), 159–185.

Holmes, J. (2003) *Power and Politeness in the Workplace.* London: Longman.

Holmes, J. (2006) *Gendered Talk at Work: Constructing Gender Identity through Workplace Discourse.* Oxford: Blackwell.

Holmes, J. (2013) *An Introduction to Sociolinguistics* (4th edn). Hoboken: Taylor and Francis.

Hopper, G. (2015) *Art, Education and Gender: The Shaping of Female Ambition.* Basingstoke: Palgrave MacMillan.

Ingersoll, J. (2003) *Evangelical Christian Women: War Stories in the Gender Battles.* New York: New York University Press.

Ivinson, G. and Murphy, P. (2007) *Rethinking Single-sex Teaching.* Toronto: Open University Press.

Ivy, D. and Backlund, P. (2008) *Gender Speak: Personal Effectiveness in Gender Communication* (4th edn). Boston: Pearson Education.

Jackson, L., Yong, Z., Witt, E., Fitzgerald, H., Von Eye, A. and Harold, R. (2009) Self-concept, self-esteem, gender, race, and information technology use. *Cyber Psychology and Behaviour* 12 (4), 437–440.

Jansz, J. and Martis, R. (2007) The Lara phenomenon: powerful female characters in video games. *Sex Roles* 56 (3/4), 141–148.

Jespersen, O. (1922) *Language: Its Nature, Development and Origin.* London: G. Allen and Unwin.

Jones, C. and Mahony, P. (eds) (1989) *Learning Our Lines: Sexuality and Social Control in Education.* London: Women's Press.

Jones, D. (1980) Gossip: Notes on women's oral culture. In C. Kramarae (ed.) *The Voices and Words of Women and Men.* Oxford: Pergamon Press.

Jones, M.G. and Wheatley, J. (2006) Gender differences in teacher-student interactions in science classrooms. *Journal of Research in Science Teaching* 27 (9), 861–874.

Jones, S.G. (1995) *Cyber Society: Computer-mediated Communication and Community.* Los Angeles: Sage.

Judd, A. (2014, 20 December) *Vancouver Park Board Votes to Install Gender-neutral Washrooms.* 11 November 2015, www.globalnews.ca.

Jule, A. (2004) *Gender and Silence in a Language Classroom: Sh-shushing the Girls*. Basingstoke, UK: Palgrave-Macmillan.

Jule, A. (2005) Language use and silence as morality: Teaching and lecturing at an evangelical theology college. In A. Jule (ed.) *Gender and the Language of Religion*. Basingstoke: Palgrave-Macmillan.

Jule, A. (ed.) (2007) *Language and Religious Identity: Women in Discourse*. Basingstoke: Palgrave Macmillan.

Jule, A. and Pedersen, B.T. (eds) (2006) *Being Feminist, Being Christian: Essays from Academia*. New York: Palgrave Macmillan.

Kendall, S. (2006) Positioning the female voice within work and family. In J. Baxter (ed.) *Speaking Out: The Female Voice in Public Contexts* (pp. 179–197). Basingstoke: Palgrave Macmillan.

Kendall, S. and Tannen, D. (1997) Gender and language in the workplace. In R. Wodak (ed.) *Gender and Discourse* (pp. 81–105). London: Sage.

Keneally, K. (2015) Julia Gillard: From Australia's first female prime minister to international superstar. *The Guardian*. 21 October.

Kilbourne, J. (2000) *Can't Buy My Love: How Advertising Changes the Way We Think and Feel*. Washington, DC: Free Press.

Kindlon, D. and Thompson, M. (1999) *Raising Cain: Protecting the Emotional Life of Boys*. New York: Ballantine Books.

Krebs, C.P., Lindquist, C.H., Warner, T.D., Fisher, B.S. and Martin, S.L. (2007) *The Campus Sexual Assault (CSA) Study*. Washington, DC: National Institute of Justice.

Labov, W. (1966). *The Social Stratification of English in New York City*. Washington: Center for Applied Linguistics.

Lacan, J. (1968) *The Language of the Self: The Function of Language in Psychoanalysis* (trans. A. Wilden). Baltimore: Johns Hopkins University Press.

Lakoff, R. (1975) *Language and Woman's Place*. New York: Harper and Row.

Lakoff, R. (1995) Cries and whispers: The shattering of silence. In K. Hall and M. Bucholtz (eds) *Gender Articulated: Language and the Socially Constructed Self* (pp. 25–50). London: Routledge.

Lakoff, R. (2004) *Language and Woman's Place: Text and Commentaries*. New York: Harper and Row.

Lazar, M. (ed.) (2005) *Feminist Critical Discourse Analysis: Studies in Gender, Power and Ideology*. London: Palgrave Macmillan.

Levy, A. (2005) *Female Chauvinist Pigs: Women and the Rise of Raunch Culture*. New York: Free Press.

Lindsay, G. and Muijs D. (2006) Challenging underachievement in boys. *Educational Research* 48 (3), 313–332.

Litosseliti, L. (2006) *Gender and Language: Theory and Practice*. London: Arnold.

Mac an Ghaill, M. (2000) The cultural production of English masculinities in late modernity. *Canadian Journal of Education* 25 (2), 88–101.

Maccoby, E.E. (1990) Gender and relationships: A developmental account. *American Psychologist* 45 (4), 513–520.

Mahony, P. (1985) *Schools for the Boys? Co-education Reassessed*. London: Hutchinson.

Maltz, D.N. and Borker, R.A. (1998) A cultural approach to male-female miscommunication. In J. Coates (ed.) *Language and Gender: A Reader* (pp. 417–434). Oxford: Blackwell.

Martino, W. (2008) Male teachers as role models: Addressing issues of masculinity, pedagogy and the re-masculinization of schooling. *Curriculum Inquiry* 38 (2), 189–223.

McConnell-Ginet, S. (2000) Breaking through the glass ceiling: Can linguistic awareness help? In J. Holmes (ed.) *Gendered Speech in Social Context: Perspectives from Gown to Town* (pp. 259–282). Wellington: Victoria University Press.

McElhinny, B. (1998) 'I don't smile much anymore.' In J. Coates (ed.) *Language and Gender: A Reader* (pp. 309–327). Oxford: Blackwell.

McElhinny, B. (2003) Ideologies of public and private language in sociolinguistics. In R. Wodak (ed.) *Gender and Discourse* (pp. 106–139). London: Sage.

McEntarter, H.K. (2016) *Navigating Gender and Sexuality in the Classroom: Narrative Insights from Students and Educators*. New York: Routledge.

McKnight, L. (2015) Still in the LEGO (LEGOS) room: Female teachers designing curriculum around girls' popular culture for the coeducational classroom in Australia. *Gender and Education* 27 (7), 909–927.

McRobbie, A. (1994) Folk devils fight back. *New Left Review* 203, 107–116.

Mernissi, F. (2002) *Islam and Democracy: Fear of the Modern World*. New York: Basic Books.

Meyerhoff, M. (2005) Forward. In A. Jule (ed.) *Gender and the Language of Religion* (pp. x–xi). Basingstoke: Palgrave MacMillan.

Mezit, L. (2011). Language, gender and religion: an investigation into some gender specific issues in religious texts and the impact of language on the role of woman in Judaism, Christianity and Islam. Master's thesis: University of Agder.

Mills, S. (2003) Third wave feminist linguistics and the analysis of sexism. *Discourse Analysis Online*, 12 March 2016. www.extra.shu.ac.uk.

Mills, S. (2012) *Gender Matters: Feminist Linguistic Analysis*. London: Equinox.

Mills, S. (ed.) (2013) *Language and Gender: Interdisciplinary Perspectives*. New York: Longman.

Mintzberg, H. (1973) *The Nature of Managerial Work*. New York: Harper & Row.

Mohler-Kuo, M., Dowdall, G., Koss, M. and Wechsler, H. (2004) Correlates of rape while intoxicated in a national sample of college women. *Journal of Studies on Alcohol* 65, 37–45.

Monckton-Smith, J. (2012) *Murder, Gender and the Media: Narratives of Dangerous Love*. Basingstoke: Palgrave.

Moran, C. (2011) *How to be a Woman*. London: Ebury Press.

Moran, C. (2016) It's the 21st century and you are not a dick. *Esquire Magazine*, p. 132.

Mullany, L. (2003) Identity and role construction: A sociolinguistic study of gender and discourse in management. Unpublished PhD thesis, Nottingham Trent University, UK.

Munford, R. (2014) *Feminism in Popular Culture*. New Brunswick, NJ: Rutgers.

Mutch, B.H. (2003) Women in the church: A North American perspective. In M. Hancock (ed.) *Christian Perspectives on Gender, Sexuality, and Community* (pp. 181–193). Vancouver, BC: Regent College Press.

Myers, G. (1998) *Ad Worlds: Brands, Media, Audiences*. London: Arnold.

National LBG&T partnership, The. www.nationallgbtpartnership.org.

Nichols, P. (1998) Black women in the rural south: Conservative and innovative. In J. Coates (ed.) *Language and Gender: A Reader* (pp. 55–63). Oxford: Blackwell.

Noon, S. (2016) *Talk Sex Today*. Kelowna, BC, Canada: Wood Lake Publishing.

Ntiri, D.W. (2015) *Literacy as Gendered Discourse: Engaging the Voices of Women in Global Societies*. Charlotte, NC: Information Age Publishers.

O'Barr, W. and Atkins, B. (1998) 'Women's language' or 'powerless language'? In J. Coates (ed.) *Language and Gender: A Reader* (pp. 377–387). Oxford: Blackwell.

O'Quinn, E.J. (2013) *Girls Literacy Experiences in and out of School: Learning and Composing Gendered Identities*. New York: Routledge.

Oakley, A. (1972) *Gender and Society*. London: Temple Smith.

Orenstein, P. (2016) *Girls and Sex: Navigating the Complicated New Landscape*. New York: Harper.

Oxford, R. (1994) La difference ... : Gender differences in a second/foreign language learning styles and strategies. In J. Sunderland (ed.) *Exploring Gender: Questions and Implications for English Language Education* (pp. 140–147). New York: Prentice Hall.

Paechter, C. (1998) *Educating the Other: Gender, Power and Schooling*. London: Falmer.

Pease, A. (2012) *Modernism, Feminism and the Culture of Boredom*. Cambridge: Cambridge University Press.

Pepe, V., Holmes, R., Annette, A., Stride, A., Mosse, M. (eds) (2015) *I Call Myself a Feminist*. London: Vivago Press.

Peters, M. (2007) The math on Miss motor mouth. *Psychology Today* March, April, 21.

Peterson, S. (2015) International/global political economy. In L.J. Shepherd (ed.) *Gender Matters in Global Politics* (pp. 173–185). London: Routledge.

Pichler, P. and Coates, J. (2011) *Language and Gender: A Reader* (2nd ed.) Hoboken, New Jersey: Wiley-Blackwell.

Pipher, M. (1994) *Reviving Ophelia: Saving the Souls of Adolescent Girls*. New York: Ballantine Books.

Plascow, J. (1990) *Standing Again at Sinai*. New York: HarperOne Publishing.

Pollack, W. (1998) *Real Boys: Rescuing our Sons from the Myths of Boyhood*. New York: Henry Holt & Co.

Rafelman, R. (1997) The party line. *Toronto Life*. November.

Rashidi, N. and Naderi, S. (2012) The effect of gender on the patterns of classroom interaction. *Education* 2 (3) 30–36.

Raymond, J. (1985) *A Passion for Friends: Towards a Philosophy of Female Affection*. Boston, MA: Beacon Press.

Redfern, C. and Aune, K. (2013) *Reclaiming the F Word: Feminism Today*. London: Zed Books.

Reskin, B. and Roos, P. (eds) (1990) *Job Queues, Gender Queues: Explaining Women's Inroads into Male Occupations*. Philadelphia: Temple University Press.

Rosin, H. (2012) *The End of Men and the Rise of Women*. London: Penguin.

Rottenberg, C. (2014) The rise of neoliberal feminism. *Cultural Studies* Vol. 28 (3) 421.

Royse, P., Lee, J., Undrahbuyan, B., Hopson, M., and Consalvo, M. (2007) Women and games: Technologies of the gendered self. *New Media & Society* 9 (4), 555–576.

Ryan, H. (10 January 2014) *What does Trans* Mean, and Where did it come From?* Slate. 16 February 2016, www.slate.com.

Sable, R., Danis, F., Mauzy, D.L. and Gallagher, S.K. (2006) Barriers to reporting sexual assault for women and men: Perspectives of college students. *Journal of American College Health* 55 (3), 157–162.

Sadker, M. and Sadker, D. (1990) Confronting sexism in the college classroom. In S. Gabriel and I. Smithson (eds) *Gender in the Classroom: Power and Pedagogy* (pp. 176–187). Chicago: University of Illinois Press.

Sales, N.J. (2016) *American Girls: Social Media and the Secret Lives of Teenagers.* New York: Knopf.

Sandberg, S. (2015) *Lean in: Women, Work and the Will to Lead.* London: Emery Publishing.

Sapir, E. (1929) The status of linguistics as a science. In D.G. Madelbaum (ed.) (1958) *Culture, Language and Personality.* Berkeley, CA: University of California Press.

Sauntson, H. (2012) *Approaches to Gender and Spoken Classroom Discourse.* Basingstoke: Palgrave.

Sauntson, H. and Kyratzis, S. (eds) (2007) *Language, Sexualities and Desires: Cross Cultural Perspectives.* Basingstoke: Palgrave.

Shapiro, E. (2010) *Gender Circuits: Bodies and Identities in a Technological Age.* New York: Routledge.

Sheldon, A. (1997) Talking power: Girls, gender enculturation and discourse. In R. Wodak (ed.) *Gender and Discourse* (pp. 225–244). London: Sage.

Shibuya, A., Sakamoto, A., Ihori, N. and Yukawa, S. (2008) The effects of the presence and contexts of video games on children: A longitudinal study in Japan. *Stimulation and Gaming* 39 (4), 528–539.

Short, G. and Carrington, B. (1990) Discourses on gender: The perspectives of children aged six and eleven. In C. Skelton (ed.) *Whatever Happens to Little Women?: Gender and Primary Schooling.* Milton Keyes: Open University Press.

Simmons, R. (2002) *Odd Girl Out: The Hidden Culture of Aggression in Girls.* Orlando, FL: Harcourt Books.

Skelton, C. and Francis, B. (eds) (2005) *A Feminist Critique of Education: 15 Years of Gender Education.* London: Routledge.

Smith, S.L. (2006a) *G Movies Give Boys a D: Portraying Males as Dominant, Disconnected and Dangerous.* Program Brief, *See Jane* Program at Dads and Daughters. May, www.SeeJane.org.

Smith, S.L. (2006b) *Where the Girls Aren't: Gender Disparity Saturates G-Rated Films.* Program Brief, *See Jane* Program at Dads and Daughters. February, www.SeeJane.org.

Smithers, R. (2016) *Boots Revises Cost of Products over Accusations of Sexist Pricing.* 3 February, www.guardian.com.

Spender, D. (1980) *Man Made Language.* London: Pandora.

Spender, D. (1982) *Invisible Women: The Schooling Scandal.* London: Writers and Readers Publishing Corp.

Spender, D. and Sarah, E. (1980) *Learning to Lose: Sexism and Education.* London: The Women's Press.

Stanworth, M. (1983) *Gender and Schooling: A Study of Sexual Divisions in the Classroom.* London: Women's Research and Resources Centre.

Stevens, K. (2006) *Gender Bias in Teacher Interactions with Students.* Master's Thesis, Dordt College, Sioux Center, Iowa.

Stoddard, C. (2015) One year after Rolling Stone's disastrous 'A Rape on Campus,' here's how University of Virginia classrooms have changed. See www.bustle.com (accessed December 18, 2015).

Sunderland, J. (1998) Girls being quiet: A problem for foreign language classrooms. *Language Teaching Research* 2.

Sunderland, J. (2004) *Gendered Discourses.* Basingstoke: Palgrave.

Swann, J. (1998) Talk control: An illustration from the classroom of problems in analysing male dominance of conversation. In J. Coates (ed.) *Language and Gender: A Reader* (pp. 185–196). Oxford: Blackwell.

Swann, J. and Graddol, D. (1995) Feminising classroom talk? In S. Mills (ed.) *Language and Gender: Interdisciplinary Perspectives* (pp. 135–148). Harlow, Essex: Addison Wesley Longman.

Szecsi, G. (2012) Mediated communities in the age of electronic communication. *KOME-Journal of Pure Communication Inquiry* 46–53.

Talbot, M. (1995) A synthetic sisterhood: False friends in a teenage magazine. In K. Hall and M. Bucholtz (eds) *Gender Articulated: Language and the Socially Constructed Self* (pp. 143–168). New York: Routledge.

Talbot, M. (1998) *Language and Gender: An Introduction.* Cambridge: Polity Press.

Talbot, M. (2010) *Language and Gender: An Introduction* (2nd edn). Cambridge: Polity Press.

Tannen, D. (1990) *You Just Don't Understand: Women and Men in Conversation.* New York: William Morrow.

Tannen, D. (1995) *Talking from 9 to 5.* London: Virago.

Tannen, D. (1998) *The Argument Culture.* London: Virago.

Thomas, L. (1996) Invisible women: Gender and the exclusive language debate. In S. Porter (ed.) *The Nature of Religious Language: A Colloquium* (pp. 159–169). Sheffield: Sheffield University Press.

Thornborrow, J. (2014) *Power Talk: Language and Interaction in Institutional Discourse.* Abingdon, Oxon: Routledge.

Today's New International Version (2002) *The Bible.* Grand Rapids, MI: Zondervan Publishing.

Totten, P. and Berbary, L. (2015) Excluded from privilege? Black American fraternity men's negotiations of hegemonic masculinity. *Leisure/Luisir* 39 (1), 37–60.

Trudgill, P. (1974) *Sociolinguistics: An Introduction*. Middlesex: Penguin.

Ulaby, N. (2008) *The Bechdel Rule: Defining Popular Culture Character*. NPR. 8 September, www.npr.org/templates/story/story.php?storyId = 94202522.

Valpy, M. (2007) Are Anglicans facing a great schism? *Globe and Mail*, March 19, A3.

Wadud, A. (2005) Citizenship and faith. In M. Friedman (ed.) *Women and Citizenship, Studies in Feminist Philosophy* (pp. 170–187). Oxford New York: Oxford University Press.

Walkerdine, V. (1990) *Schoolgirl Fictions*. London: Versco.

Walsh, C. (2001) *Gender and Discourse: Language and Power in Politics, the Church and Organizations*. London: Pearson Education.

Wesleyan University creates all-inclusive acronym: LBTTQQFAGPBNSM. *This Week*. 15 February 2015, www.theweek.com/speedreads/541158/wesleyan-university-creates-allinclusive-acronym-lbttqqfagpbdsm.

West, C. (1990) Not just 'doctors' orders': Directive-response sequences in patients' visits to women and men physicians. *Discourse and Society* ICI, 85–112.

Westwood, R. (2016) In the age of sexting, feminism is the anti-chill for teens. And that is chilling. In *Vancouver Metro*, online. March 20.

Wichterich, C. (2000) *The Globalized Woman: Reports from a Future of Inequality*. New York: Zed Books.

Williams, D. and Skoric, M. (2005) Internet fantasy violence: A test of aggression in an online game. *Communication Monographs* 72 (2), 217–233.

Williams, D., Martins, N., Consalvo, M. and Ivory, J. (2009) The virtual census: representations of gender, race and age in video games. *New Media and Society* 11 (5), 815–834.

Wilson, G. (2014) *Your Brain on Porn: Internet Pornography and the Emerging Science of Addiction*. Taiwan: Commonwealth Publishing.

Wiseman, R. (2002) *Queen Bees and Wannabees: Helping Your Daughter Survive Gossip, Boyfriends, and Other Realities of Adolescence*. New York: Crown Publishers.

Wodak, R. (ed.) (1997) *Gender and Discourse*. London: Sage.

Women's Media: The Site for Working Women (2003) www.womensmedia.com.

Wood, J. (1997) Clarifying the issues. *Personal Relationships* 4 (3), 221–228.

Wood, J. (2013) *Gendered Lives: Communication, Gender and Culture* (10th edn). Boston: Wadsworth.

Woolf, V. (1928) *A Room of One's Own*. London: Penguin.

World Health Organization, Neo-liberal Ideas www.who.int/goverance/eb/who.

Zayzafoon, L. (2005) *The Production of the Muslim Woman: Negotiating Text, History and Ideology*. Lemington: Lemington Books.

Zimbardo, P. and Coulombe, N. (2016) *Man, Interrupted: Why Young Men are Struggling and What We Can Do about It*. Newburyport, MA: Conari Press.

Zorrila, M.G. (2013) Public relations challenges: Opinion leaders and video games. Master's Thesis, Radford University.

Index

. . . .

Headings in italics refer to publications or campaigns.

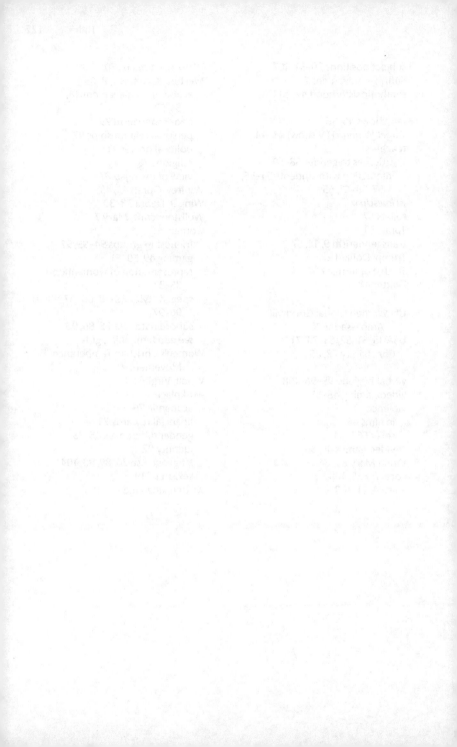